MANUAL
of
ARTICULATION
and
PHONOLOGICAL
DISORDERS

Infancy Through Adulthood

Clinical Competence Series

Series Editor
Robert T. Wertz, Ph.D.

MANUAL
of
ARTICULATION
and
PHONOLOGICAL
DISORDERS

Infancy through Adulthood

Ken M. Bleile, Ph.D.

SINGULAR PUBLISHING GROUP, INC.
SAN DIEGO · LONDON

Singular Publishing Group, Inc.
401 West "A" Street, Suite 325
San Diego, California 92101-7904

Singular Publishing Ltd.
19 Compton Terrace
London, N1 2UN, UK

e-mail: singpub@mail.cerfnet.com
Website: http://www.singpub.com

© 1995 by Singular Publishing Group, Inc.
Second Printing August 1997

Typeset in 10/12 Times by CFW Graphics
Printed in the United States of America by McNaughton & Gunn

Library of Congress Cataloging-in-Publication Data

Bleile, Kenneth Mitchell.
    Manual of articulation and phonological disorders. Infancy
through adulthood / by Ken M. Bleile.
        p.   cm. — (Clinical competence series)
    Includes bibliographical references and index.
    ISBN 1–56593–343–5
    1. Articulation disorders. 2. I. Title.
II. Series.
        [DNLM: 1. Articulation Disorders — diagnosis. 2. Articulation
Disorders — therapy. 3. Voice Disorders — diagnosis. 4. Voice
Disorders — therapy.   WM 475 8646m 1994]
RC424.7.856   1994
616.85'5 — dc20
DNLM/DLC
for Library of Congress   94-31970
                                                                    CIP

CONTENTS

LIST OF APPENDIXES

FOREWORD

com·pe·tence (kom'pǝ tǝns) n. The state or quality
of being properly or well qualified; capable.

Clinicians crave competence. They pursue it through education and experience, through emulation and innovation. Some are more successful than
others in attaining what they seek. Fortunately, we have colleagues who
assist us. Dr. Ken M. Bleile is one of those. His effort, *Manual of Articulation
and Phonological Disorders: Infancy Through Adulthood,* is one of several
books in the Singular Clinical Competence Series. It is designed to move
each of us further along the path that leads to clinical competence. Dr.
Bleile introduces us to the terminology, tells us how to screen and appraise,
leads us through the analysis of screening and appraisal data, presents
treatment principles, and lists facilitative techniques designed to achieve
the desired results. He is a skilled investigator and a competent clinician,
and his book conveys what makes him that way. Dr. Bleile reaches across
generations — from old timers who grew up when there were only articulation disorders to recent graduates whose academic preparation emphasized
phonological disorders. He creates order out of material that can be confusing, and he demonstrates how what is known can be put into productive
practice. Indeed, we are fortunate to have colleagues like Ken Bleile who
have "been there, done that, and do it very well." Your attention to what he
provides indicates your competence and your effort to improve it, because
competent clinicians seek competence as much for what it demands as for
what it promises.

Robert T. Wertz, Ph.D.
Series Editor

PREFACE

Clients with articulation and phonological disorders span the age range, from infants and toddlers to preschoolers, school-age children, and adults. Some clients have problems in speech as their only disability; more often, however, a client's difficulty in speech is embedded in other developmental and medical problems, especially among the younger populations just now beginning to appear in the case loads of many clinicians. The settings of care for clients with articulation and phonological disorders include schools and preschools, hospitals, early intervention programs, and the home.

This book was written to serve as a clinical resource for the care of clients of all ages and levels of severity. I hope the manual will serve as a compendium of materials and practical ideas for clinicians who wish to consider a range of clinical options, selecting those that seem good and discarding those that appear less appropriate. I hope students will find the manual a readable introduction to some complicated concepts and issues, and that it will serve as a beginning point to explore original research papers and monographs on articulation and phonological disorders.

The book is organized into six chapters. Chapter 1 addresses issues that arise prior to beginning care, including definitions of speech disorders, the legal basis for provision of care, medical precautions, notational conventions, transcription symbols, and specialized terminology. Chapter 2 describes options in nonstandardized and standardized screenings and complete assessments. The chapter concludes with appendixes of forms designed for use in clinical settings.

Chapter 3 presents the most widely accepted options in articulation and phonological analysis. Major topics include measures to assess severity and intelligibility; age norms to assess prespeech vocalizations, phonetic inventories, error patterns, and consonants and consonant clusters; better abilities to assess stimulability, key environments, key words, and responsiveness to phonetic placement and shaping techniques; and related analyses to determine adjusted and developmental age, the influence of dialect, and acquisition strategies. The chapter concludes with appendixes designed to assist clinicians in performing the major analyses described in the chapter.

Chapters 4 and 5 describe treatment principles and procedures, respectively. The major topics discussed in Chapter 4 include the purposes of treatment at four stages in articulation and phonological development; selection of long- and short-term goals, treatment targets, number of treatment targets, criteria for changing treatment targets, linguistic level and phonetic environments in which to introduce treatment targets; summaries of published treatment programs; and assessing treatment progress. Chapter 5 describes techniques designed to facilitate articulation and phonological development, including bombardment, metaphors, descriptions and demonstrations, touch cues, contrast therapy, building syllables and words, facilitative talk, and direct instruction. Chapter 5 concludes with extensive appendixes focusing on descriptions and demonstrations, word pairs, and phonetic placement and shaping techniques.

The book concludes with Chapter 6, which summarizes the major care options for clients with articulation and phonological disorders.

ACKNOWLEDGMENTS

I wish to thank the clients whom I have had the pleasure to treat during my long and ongoing apprenticeship in the study of articulation and phonological disorders. I also wish to thank the Division of Speech Pathology and Audiology at the University of Hawaii for its support and encouragement. Most especially, I want to thank the students in articulation and phonology courses at the University of Hawaii who shared generously of their time and ideas during the year over which this book was written. My special thanks also go to Barbara Bernhardt and Ann Tyler for their insightful reviews of early drafts of this manuscript, and to Jolynn Vannucci and Sandy Walsh for contributing appendixes to this book. Finally, I wish to thank Terry and Judy for making home such an enjoyable place to be.

For Judy

And in Memory of Charles Van Riper

CHAPTER

1

Orientation

The following topics are discussed in this chapter:

I. CHAPTER OVERVIEW

The sections in this chapter address the following basic questions: What are articulation and phonological disorders? How are articulation and phonological disorders distinguished from other types of speech problems? What is the legal basis for providing care? What safety precautions should be followed with clients with medical needs? What specialized terminology and notations are encountered in the care of clients with articulation and phonological disorders? The chapter concludes with an appendix that provides a complete set of diacritics for American English consonants and vowels.

II. ARTICULATION AND PHONOLOGICAL DISORDERS

Speech has a dual nature. It is a motor skill requiring the most rapid and skilled movements the human body is able to perform, and it is the primary channel through which human language is realized. Virtually everyone agrees that speech disorders may arise from problems in either speech motor control (articulation disorders) or language knowledge (phonological disorders), even though research has not yet provided the means to make this differential diagnosis in clinical practice.

C. Terminology

The topic of this book is a certain type of speech problem. In recognition of the dual nature of speech, these speech problems are called **articulation and phonological disorders.** This terminology is used by many authors (Bernthal & Bankson, 1993; Creaghead, Newman, & Secord, 1989; Lowe, 1994; Weiss, Gordon, & Lillywhite, 1987), but differs from that used by others, who prefer either the term **articulation disorder** or **phonological disorder** to encompass both problems in speech motor control (articulation) and language (phonology) (Fey, 1992; Hoffman, Schuckers, & Daniloff, 1989; Hodson, 1994; Locke, 1983a; Shriberg & Kwiatkowski, 1982; Shelton & McReynolds, 1979; Winitz, 1984). Use of "articulation disorder" as the sole term is intended to emphasize that speech is a motor activity, whereas use of "phonological disorder" as the sole term is intended to emphasize that speech requires knowledge of language. Additional terminology the reader may encounter, which means approximately what is referred to here as articulation and phonological disorders, includes functional speech disorder, developmental speech disorder, phonomotor disorder, speech disorder, functional articulation disorder, and — more rarely — idiopathic speech disorder. Finally, some authors, noting that persons with articulation and phonological disorders often speak similarly to younger children without speech problems, prefer to use the term delay rather than disorder (Curtiss, Katz, & Tallal, 1992; Leonard, 1985).

B. Stages

It is often convenient to have some means of describing aspects of care that change according to the client's level of articulation and phonological development. For this reason, the discussion of articulation and phonological development that follows is divided into four broad stages. The primary articulation and phonological characteristics of the four stages are summarized in Table 1–1 and described below.

1. **Stage 1.** This stage occurs in typically developing infants from birth to approximately 12 months of age. During this stage vocalizations are seldom, if ever, used for referential purposes. Activities such as cooing and babbling allow the client to "practice the vocal mechanism." Articulation and phonological care focuses primarily on facilitating the acquisition of vocal skills that underlie later speech development.

2. **Stage 2.** This stage occurs in typically developing toddlers from approximately 12 to 24 months of age. During this stage speech gradually comes to replace eye contact, gestures, and vocalizations as the primary means of communication as the

Table 1–1. Primary purposes of care at four stages in articulation and phonological development.

Stages	Age Range in Typically Developing Children	Primary Purpose of Care
Stage 1	0–12 ms	Facilitate practice of vocal skills that serve as the basis for later speech development
Stage 2	12–24 ms	Facilitate the acquisition of sounds and syllables in specific words
Stage 3	2–5 yrs	Facilitate the elimination of errors affecting classes of sounds
Stage 4	5 yrs and older	Facilitate the elimination of errors affecting late-acquired consonants, consonant clusters, and unstressed syllables in more difficult multisyllabic words

---

Stages

Stages provide a useful shorthand. It is quicker, for example, to say "clients in Stage 3" than it is to say "clients with errors affecting sound classes and who have expressive vocabularies over 100 different words." Importantly, the stages used in this book refer to a level that corresponds to a client's articulation and phonological development — this may or may not be the same as the client's chronological age. (Procedures to determine the age level most closely corresponding to the client's level of articulation and phonological development are described in Chapter 3.) For example, a school-aged child in Stage 3 receives treatment using principles developed to treat clients whose speech contains errors affecting sound classes. Naturally, specific treatment activities are selected based on the client's interests rather than level of articulation and phonological development. An adult in Stage 4, for example, receives treatment using principles developed to treat clients with errors affecting a few late-acquired consonants, consonant clusters, and unstressed syllables in more difficult multisyllabic words although the particular activities and instructions used would be modified to reflect the interests of an adult.

---

client develops a small expressive vocabulary (typically less than 100 words by 24 months of age in typically developing toddlers) to express his or her thoughts, feelings, and needs. Articulation and phonological care focuses primarily on facilitating the acquisition of sounds and syllables in specific words.

3. **Stage 3.** This stage occurs in typically developing preschoolers from approximately 2 to 5 years of age. Speech is well-established by the beginning of this stage, although the client continues to experience difficulty in pronouncing entire sound classes. Articulation and phonological care focuses primarily on eliminating errors affecting classes of sounds.

4. **Stage 4.** This stage occurs in typically developing school-aged children aged approximately 5 years and older. During this

stage the client's speech is similar to that of his or her community, although errors on late-acquired consonants, consonant clusters, and unstressed syllables in more difficult multisyllabic words may still occur. Articulation and phonological care focuses primarily on eliminating errors affecting individual consonants and consonant clusters and on producing unstressed syllables in more difficult multisyllabic words.

A Lexical Approach

A major difference between treating clients in Stage 2 and Stage 3 lies in emphasis. For clients in Stage 2, the emphasis is on using sounds and syllables to facilitate word acquisition, whereas for clients in Stage 3 the emphasis is on using words to facilitate sound and syllable acquisition (Bleile, in press; Bleile & Miller, 1994). The word is given a central role in the treatment of clients in Stage 2 based on research that indicates that expressive vocabulary development (words actually used for communication, rather than simply words the client understands) is a primary means through which younger children acquire the rules of speech and language (Ferguson & Farwell, 1975). Articulation and phonological problems are also thought to be major factors in limiting expressive vocabulary development in several clinical populations (Miller, 1992; Paul, 1991). For these reasons, a lexical approach to treating clients in Stage 2 is emphasized in this book as a means of using articulation and phonological principles to facilitate expressive vocabulary development.

C. Characteristics of Articulation and Phonological Disorders

Not all speech problems are articulation and phonological disorders. A laryngeal anomaly, for example, may result in significant difficulties in speech motor control, but is not the type of difficulty that is amenable to the treatment principles described in this book. The types of **speech problems** addressed in this book **meet four criteria:**

The speech is not directly attributable to physical damage to the speech mechanism, sensory systems, peripheral nervous system, or central nervous system.

The speech is similar to that of children without articulation and phonological disorders.

The speech is not the result of dialect.

The speech is considered disordered either by the client and/or members of the client's community.

1. **First and Second Criteria.** The first and second criteria distinguish articulation and phonological disorders from speech problems arising directly from physical difficulties such as cranial nerve damage, unrepaired cleft palate, laryngeal anomalies, or difficulties in respiratory control. These criteria do not exclude from consideration articulation and phonological disorders that occur in addition to problems arising from physical difficulties, nor do they exclude compensatory speech adjustments that persons with physical disabilities often develop, which are often amenable to remediation using articulation and phonological principles.

2. **Third and Fourth Criteria.** The third criterion distinguishes articulation and phonological disorders from dialect differences. The former signify difficulties in speech motor and language learning; the latter are part of the language system of the client's community. For this reason, although dialect can be reduced using articulation and phonological principles, dialect itself is not considered a type of articulation and phonological disorder. The fourth criterion recognizes that cultures and ethnic groups may differ both in what they identify as articulation and phonological disorders and in the priority they assign to remediating various types of articulation and phonological disorders (Bleile & Wallach, 1992; Taylor & Peters-Johnson, 1986).

D. Prevalence

An articulation and phonological disorder is a type of communication disorder and may occur as either an isolated developmental problem or as part of a larger constellation of difficulties, including language disorders, mental retardation, respiratory problems, neurological injuries, cerebral palsy, and oro-facial anomalies.

1. **Prevalence of Communication Disorders.** The following are prevalence statistics for communication disorders.

    a. **Comparison to Other Disabilities.** The most commonly diagnosed handicapping condition among persons aged 6 to 21 years is learning disability (47.7%), followed by communication disorders (23.1%), mental retardation (13.9%), and emotional disturbance (9%) (U.S. Department of Education, 1990).

    b. **Age.** Nearly 2% of persons under 18 years old have communication disorders. This number drops to below 1% of the population between 18 and 64 years old and then rises above 1% for persons 64 years and older (Schoenborn & Marano, 1989).

    c. **Gender and Race.** Males younger than 45 years old are almost twice as likely to have communication disorders as females. African-Americans younger than 45 years old are almost one third more likely to be diagnosed as having communication disorders as Caucasians (Schoenborn & Marano, 1989).

    d. **Socioeconomic Scale.** Persons younger than 45 years old living in families making less than $10,000 annually are approximately twice as likely to be diagnosed as having communication disorders as peers living in homes making between $20,000 to $34,999 annually (Schoenborn & Marano, 1989).

    e. **Educational Setting.** Nearly 75% of all school-aged children with communication disorders receive their education in a regular classroom setting (U.S. Department of Education, 1990).

2. **Prevalence of Articulation and Phonological Disorders.** The following are prevalence statistics for articulation and phonological disorders.

    a. **Compared to Other Communication Disorders.** Approximately 32% of all communication disorders are articulation and phonological disorders (Slater, 1992).

    b. **Language Disorders.** Approximately 75% to 85% of preschoolers with articulation and phonological disorders also experience disorders in language (Shriberg & Kwiat-kowski, 1988; Paul & Shriberg, 1982).

c. **Clinician Exposure.** Approximately 92% of clinicians have clients with articulation and phonological disorders on their caseloads (Shewan, 1988).

E. Legal Basis of Care

Clinical care for articulation and phonological disorders is provided under a variety of local, state, and national laws. The two most pertinent pieces of federal legislation are **Public Law 99-457** (PL 99-457), The Education of Handicapped Act Amendments, and **Public Law 94-142 (PL 94-142),** The Education for All Handicapped Children (Kitley & Buzby-Hadden, 1993).

A New Clinical Frontier

Passage and enactment of Public Law 99-457 has helped to create a new clinical frontier: articulation and phonological care of clients in Stage 1 and Stage 2. One hope in writing about these clients is to encourage other clinicians and researchers to explore how best to serve our younger and more developmentally at-risk populations.

---

1. **PL 99-457.** Part H of PL 99-457 applies to children 0–2 years and has been extended by most states to children up to 3 years old. PL 99-457 provides legal protection to (1) children with developmental delays in cognition, physical skills, communication, or psychosocial development and (2) children with physical or mental conditions that place them at a high probability for future developmental delays, including fetal alcohol syndrome, seizure disorders, and chromosonal abnormalities such as Down syndrome. The law gives individual states discretion to decide whether to develop laws to protect children with other conditions that place them at-risk for future developmental difficulties, including very low birth weight resulting from prematurity, respiratory distress, and asphyxia.

2. **PL 94-142.** PL 94-142 mandates free and appropriate education to all children with handicaps aged 3 through 21 years.

Appropriate education includes a thorough assessment to determine the nature and degree of disability, education tailored to the individual needs of children, placement in the least restrictive environment, and provision of supplementary services to help ensure the success of programs for each child.

F. Safety Precautions for Clients with Medical Needs

Prior to providing services to any client with an articulation and phonological disorder, speech-language clinicians must be knowledgeable about basic safety procedures, including cardiopulmonary resuscitation (CPR). Additionally, speech-language clinicians working with clients with medical needs must be well versed in the safety procedures for the populations with which they come into contact. The following safety precaution guidelines are adapted from Bleile (in press). Readers interested in more information on medical issues affecting persons with developmental disabilities are referred to Batshaw (1992) and, for children with tracheostomies, Bleile (1993a).

1. **Infection Control Guidelines.** Basic infection control guidelines should be followed when providing care to all clients with medical needs.

   a. **Hand Washing.** Many persons with medical needs have relatively weak immune systems, and diseases carried by staff are a primary source of infection. The most effective means of reducing spread of infection is through careful washing after each client. Other times when hand washing should be performed are when coming on or off duty, when the hands are dirty, after toilet use, after blowing or wiping one's nose, after handling client secretions, and on completion of duty.

   To wash, wet the hands and forearms, apply soap, and wash all areas of the hands and forearms for 1 to 2 minutes, being careful to wash nail beds and between the fingers. Afterwards, rinse the soap from your hands and forearms thoroughly. Use an unused paper towel to turn off the water faucet, and then discard the paper towel.

   b. **Toy Washing.** Toys are a possible source of infection for children with medical needs, because children may place toys in their mouths, or may put their fingers in their mouths or noses after playing with an infected toy. Wear gloves to clean possibly infected toys. Wipe each toy with warm, soapy water and then rinse. Next, spray or wipe each toy with a disinfectant such as 1:10 solution of household bleach. Finally, rinse the toy well and air dry for 10 minutes.

Clients with Medical Needs

At first, persons new to working with persons with medical needs may find that following medical safety precautions imposes a barrier between establishing a relaxed, natural rapport with the client (Bleile, in press). After some time to adjust, however, clinicians usually report that the client's medical needs cease to dominate their attention and they are able to interact with the client confident that they are providing care safely.

---

2. **Physiological Warning Signs.** Clients with medical conditions sometimes experience sudden, even life-threatening, changes in their medical status. Clinicians who work with these clients must be able to recognize and respond appropriately to emergency situations if they occur. The most common physiological warning signs (or Red Flags) associated with six possibly life-threatening conditions are discussed below. If the warning signs are observed, the clinician should immediately contact the staff member (typically a physician or nurse) designated to handle medical problems.

   a. **Mechanical ventilation.** Mechanical ventilation is provided through a machine that breathes in and out for the client. The primary indicator for mechanical ventilation in children is broncho pulmonary dysplasia (Bleile, 1993b; Metz, 1993). The physiological warning signs most commonly encountered in clients receiving mechanical ventilation include changes in skin color, exaggerated breathing, coughing, alteration in heart rate or respiratory rate, and either lethargy or irritability.

b. Tracheostomy. Tracheostomy is a surgical opening below the larynx on the anterior neck (Handler, 1993). Persons with tracheostomy assistance breathe through a hole (stoma) placed in the anterior neck. The most common daily hazards associated with tracheostomy care involve blockages that make breathing difficult or impossible. The physiological warning signs of blockage include a blue tint around the lips or nail beds, flared nostrils, fast breathing, a rattling noise during breathing, mucous bubbles around the tracheostomy site, coughing or gagging, clammy skin, restlessness, and either lethargy or irritability.

c. Seizures. A seizure is a type of abnormal electrical discharge from the neurons in the cortex. Physiological warning signs associated with seizures include pallor, irritability, staring, nystagmus, changes in muscle tone, and vomiting.

d. Shunt. A shunt is a device that diverts cerebrospinal fluid from a brain ventricle to another part of the body where the fluid is then absorbed. Shunts are used for persons with hydrocephalus, a condition in which excess fluid causes ventricles in the brain to become enlarged. Physiological warning signs suggesting a shunt malfunction include headaches, vomiting, lethargy, and bulging fontanel (the soft spot on the heads of infants and toddlers).

e. Gastrointestinal conditions. Gastrointestinal conditions involve problems in one or more of three areas: controlled movement of food through the body, digestion of food, and absorption of nutrients (Silverman McGowan, Kerwin, & Bleile, 1993). If a person cannot receive enough nourishment by mouth (per oral) to sustain life and continued growth, he or she is fed via a gastrostomy or jejunal tube placed into the stomach or small intestine, respectively. Physiological warning signs of problems with a gastrostomy or jejunal tube include the presence of formula leaking from the tube at either the clamp or skin site, in and out movement of the tube, increased irritability, and emesis.

f. Cardiac conditions. Cardiac conditions are medical problems affecting the heart. They may occur as isolated medical problems or in conjunction with other disabilities. Physiological warning signs associated with cardiac conditions include changes in skin color, increased heart and/or respiratory rate, chest retractions, nasal flaring, and either lethargy or irritability.

III. SPECIAL SYMBOLS AND TECHNICAL TERMINOLOGY

Extensive use of special symbols and notations in clinical practice is rare, and their use has generally been avoided in this book. Still, some special symbols, notations, and terminology are necessary; and others, although not necessary, are extremely convenient

A. Phonetic Symbols

The symbols used to transcribe American English consonants and vowels are listed in Tables 1-2 and 1-3, respectively (International Clinical Phonetics and Linguistic Association, 1992). For convenience, the American English central liquid is transcribed as [r], and the [i] and [u] vowels (which are often pronounced as diphthongs) are transcribed as [i] and [u], respectively. The consonant chart divides sounds according to place and manner, voiced/voiceless, nasal/oral, and central/lateral. The vowel chart divides sounds according to place, height, spread/unspread, and round/unround.

B. Special Symbols and Diacritics

Special symbols are used for non-English consonants and vowels. Diacritics are modifications made to symbols to describe phonetic details. The special symbols and diacritics encountered most frequently in the clinical care of articulation and phonological disorders are listed in Appendix 1A.

C. Notations

Notations offer a convenient "shorthand" way to describe speech.

1. [ ] **and / /.** Square brackets indicate a phonetic transcription, and slashes indicate a phonemic transcription. Single sounds, groups of sounds, and entire words or phrases can be placed within brackets or slashes. The following examples demonstrate the use of this notation:

Table 1-2. American English consonants.

Manner of Production	Place of Production							
	Bilabial	Labiodental	Interdental	Alveolar	Postalveolar	Palatal	Velar	Glottal
Stop								
Oral	p b			t d			k g	
Nasal	m			n			ŋ	
Fricative		f v	θ ð	s z	ʃ ʒ			h
Affricate					tʃ dʒ			
Liquid								
Central				r				
Lateral				l				
Glide	w					j		

Table 1–3. American English vowels and dipthongs.

	Place			
	Front		Back	
Height	+ Sprd[a]	Central	– Rnd[b]	+ Rnd
Close	i			u
	ɪ		ʊ	
Close mid	eɪ			oʊ
		ə		
Open mid	ɛ		ʌ	ɔ
	æ			
Open		a		ɑ

[a] = Sprd = lips spread
[b] = – Rnd = lips unrounded
     + Rnd = lips unrounded

Notes:
[ɔɪ] = tongue begins as for [ɔ] and moves toward [ɪ]
[aɪ] = tongue begins as for [a] and moves toward [ɪ]
[aʊ] = tongue begins as for [a] and moves toward [ʊ]
[ɚ] = tongue shape has both [ə]-like and [r]-like qualities

a. **Example:** The consonant "b" as in bet.
   Notation: [b] or /b/

b. **Example:** The American English voiceless stops.
   Notation: [p t k] or /p t k/

c. **Example:** The word deep.
   Notation: [dip] or /dip/

Brackets or Slashes?

I typically transcribe a client's speech within square brackets (e.g., "bee" as [bi]). Square brackets imply nothing about the phonological status of the sounds being transcribed, whereas slashes (e.g., "bee" as /bi/) indicate that the sounds being transcribed are phonemes — that is, the sounds can distinguish between words in the client's speech, just as "p" and "b" do in adult English "pea" and "bee." Determining which sounds are phonemes in a client's speech is a controversial procedure that is seldom performed in most clinical settings. For this reason, unless a phonemic analysis of the client's speech has been performed, I enclose a transcription in square brackets rather than slashes.

2. **x → y and x/y.** The literal meaning of the first notation is "x becomes y"; the literal meaning of the second notation is "x for y." Both notations provide simple ways to describe speech changes. The arrow is used most often in linguistically oriented approaches, and the slash is used in more traditional approaches. The following examples demonstrate how these notations are used:

a. **Example:** The client says [w] for [r].
Notation: r → w or w/r

b. **Example:** The client says fricatives as stops.
Notation: fricatives → stops or fricatives/stops

c. **Example:** The client deletes both members of consonant clusters.
Notation: CC → ø or ø/CC

3. **x → y/z.** This algebraic-looking notation literally means "x becomes y in the environment of z." The notation is used to describe how a phonetic or word environment affects production of speech. The "x" and "y" can be any articulation and phonological unit — features, consonants, vowels, individual sounds, syllables, or stress. The "z" typically is a distinctive feature, consonant, vowel, a syllable boundary (symbolized as "$"), or a word boundary (symbolized as "#"). The following examples demonstrate the use of this notation:

a. **Example:** The client says liquids as glides in the beginning of words.
Notation: liquids → glides/#____

b. Example: The client says [s] as [z] between vowels.
Notation: s → z/V___V

c. Example: The client says [g] as [k] at the end of syllables.
Notation: g → k/___S

d. Example: The client deletes the first member of a consonant cluster in the beginning of words.
Notation: CC → øC/#___

American English More or Less

I made an effort throughout the book to write "American English" rather than "English," because the varieties of English are too numerous for any one type of speech to serve as the standard for the rest. However, it would have been more accurate to write that the speech described in this book is "an American English." The American English spoken in Hawaii, for example, sounds vastly different from that spoken in Georgia or Vermont. Different ethnic and racial groups within the same geographical location add to the fascinating complexity of American speech.

D. Specialized Terminology

The following terminology is commonly used to describe the speech of clients with articulation and phonological disorders. Topics are abbreviations, characteristics of speech, descriptions of errors, error patterns, influence of one sound on another, manner of production, names for sounds, phonetic and word environments, place of production, prespeech and early speech, theoretical constructs, and vowels. Definitions of terms are provided after all the topics are listed.

1. Topics

a. Abbreviations

C	CVC	V
CV	S	

b. Characteristics of Speech

Aspiration

Blends

Cognates

Consonant

Consonant cluster

Dark [l]

Dentalized

Dialect

Distinctive features

Eggressive

Homorganic

Homonyms

Humped [r] and [ɚ]

Ingressive

Intonation

Lip rounding

Lips spread

Light [l]

Multisylabic

Nasality

Primary stress

Prosody

Retroflex [r] and [ɚ]

Rounding

Singleton

Spreading

Unaspirated

Velarized [l]

Voiced

Voiceless

Voicing

c. Descriptions of Errors

Apraxia

Articulation error

Articulation disorder

Brackets

Broad transcription

Buccal (pronounced "buckle") speech

Deletion

Devoicing

Diacritics

Distortion

Dysarthria

Initial consonant deletion

Lablalization

Lateral [s]

Narrow transcription

Nasalization

Omission
Pharyngeal fricative
Phonemic transcription
Phonetic transcription
Phonological error
Phonological patterns
Phonological processes
Phonological rule
Slashes
Stimulability
Stridency deletion
Substitution

d. Error Patterns

Affrication
Backing
Cluster reduction
Denasalization
Epenthesis (ePENthesis)
Final consonant deletion
Final consonant devoicing
Frontal lisp
Fronting
Gliding
Glottal replacement
Labial assimilation

Lateralization
Lateral lisp
Lisping
Metathesis (MeTAthesis)
Prevocalic voicing
Reduplication
Stopping
Syllable deletion
Velar assimilation
Vocalization
Vowel neutralization

e. Influence of One Sound on Another

Assimilation
Coalescence

Progressive assimilation
Regressive assimilation

f. Manner of Production

Affricate
Approximant

Central
Continuants

Fricative	Obstruent
Glide	Oral stop
Lateral	Semivowels
Liquid	Sibilant
Manner of production	Sonorants
Nasals	Stop
Nasal stop	Strident

g. Names for Sounds

Capital "E"	Long "s" Open "o"
Caret	Print "a"
Digraph	Schwa
Epsilon	Theta
Horse shoe	Thorn

h. Phonetic and Word Environments

Ambisyllabic	Phonetic environments
Arrestor	Postvocalic
Environments	Resyllabification
Initial sound	Syllable initial position
Intervocalic	Syllable final position
Medial sound	Word-final position
Onset	Word-initial position
Open syllable	Word-medial position

i. Place of Production

Alveolar	Labiodental
Bilabial	Palatal
Dental	Place of production
Glottal	Postalveolar
Interdental	Velar
Labial	

j. Prespeech and Early Speech

Babble   Nonreduplicated babbling
Canonical babbling   Reduplicated babbling
Cooing   Variegated babbling
Jargon

k. Theoretical Constructs

Allophone   Phoneme
Coarticulation   Phonetics
Complementary distribution   Phonological knowledge
Discrimination training   Phonology
Independent analysis   Phonotactics
Maximal pair   Perception training
Metalinguistics   Relational analysis
Minimal pair   Rime/rhyme
Noncontrastive   Word pairs
Phone

l. Vowels

Back vowels and diphthongs   Neutral vowels
Central vowels   Open
Close   Open-mid
Close-mid   Pure vowel
Diphthong   R-colored vowel
Front vowels   Rhotic vowel
High vowels   Vowel

2. Definitions

Affricate. A consonant with a stop onset and fricative release. The American English affricates are [tʃ] and [dʒ].

Affrication. An error pattern in which stops or fricatives are pronounced as affricates; for example, "see" is pronounced as [tsi].

Allophone. A variant of a phoneme that does not affect meaning; for example, unaspirated [p⁰] and aspirated [pʰ] are allophones of the phoneme /p/.

Alveolar. A class of consonants produced with constriction between articulators at the alveolar ridge, which lies immediately posterior to the upper front teeth. The American English alveolar consonants are [t], [d], [s], [z], [n], [l], and [r].

Ambisyllabic. A consonant sometimes considered to belong to two syllables; for example, some investigators consider the second [m] in "mama" to be ambisylabic.

Approximant. Liquids and glides. The American English approximants are [l], [r], [j], and [w].

Apraxia. A disorder involving voluntary, but not involuntary, speech movements. For example, a client with apraxia may not be able to respond correctly when asked to touch the lip with the tongue but when eating may lick a crumb from the lip.

Arrestor. A consonant occurring after a vowel in the same syllable; for example, "t" is the arrestor consonant in "bit."

Articulation error. A speech error resulting from problems in speech motor control.

Articulation disorder. As defined in this book, an articulation disorder results from problems in speech motor control. Some authors use the term articulation disorder to refer to problems in both phonology and speech motor control.

Aspiration. A burst of air arising after the release of a voiceless stop in positions such as the beginning of a word; for example, in American English [t] in "tube" [tʰub].

Assimilation. The influence of one sound on another. See also **Progressive assimilation** and **Regressive assimilation**.

Babble. A prespeech vocalization in which repetitions of syllables predominate.

Backing. An error pattern in which alveolar consonants are replaced by velar consonants; for example, "tee" is pronounced as [ki].

Back vowels and diphthongs. Vowels in which the back of the tongue is the major articulator; The American English back vowels diphthongs are [u], [ʊ], [oʊ], [ɔ], [ɔɪ], [ʌ], and [ɑ].

Bilabial. Consonants made using the two lips. The American English bilabial consonants are [p], [b], [m], and [w].

Blends. Consonant clusters.

Brackets. Transcriptions enclosed by brackets indicate that the sounds were produced; no claim is made regarding whether or not the sounds are phonemes of the language. For example, placing "b" within brackets (i.e., [b]) indicates the sound was produced, but does not indicate whether or not [b] is a phoneme. See **Phoneme.**

Broad transcription. Transcription of phonemes. Broad transcriptions are enclosed within slashes. See **Phoneme** and **Slashes.**

Buccal (pronounced "buckle") speech. Speech produced by trapping air between the cheeks; sometimes called "Donald Duck speech." Children with tracheostomies often discover they can make words and short phrases using buccal speech.

C. Consonant.

Canonical babbling. See **Reduplicated babbling.**

Capital "E" (pronounced [i]). The name for the sound transcribed [ɪ].

Caret. The name for the sound transcribed [ʌ].

Central. Sounds made with air flowing over the tongue midline. All the American English consonants are central, except [l], which is lateral.

Central vowel. Vowel in which the tongue blade is the major articulator. The American English central vowel is [ə].

Close. Vowels and diphthongs produced with the tongue raised toward the roof of the mouth. The category close replaces high in the revised International Phonetic Alphabet (International Clinical Phonetics and Linguistic Association, 1992). The American English close vowels and diphthongs are [i], [ɪ], [u], and [ʊ].

Close-mid. Vowels and diphthongs produced with the tongue in a relatively neutral position. The category close-mid replaces mid in the revised International Phonetic Alphabet (International Clinical Phonetics and Linguistic Association, 1992). The American English close-mid vowels and diphthongs are [eɪ], [oʊ], and [ə].

Cluster Reduction. An error pattern in which a consonant or consonants in a consonant cluster are deleted; for example, "speed" is pronounced as [pid] or [sid].

Coalescence. The merger of two or more sounds; for example, the pronunciation of [sp] in "spy" as [f], which appears be a coalescence of the place of production of [p] (labial) and the manner of production of [s] (fricative).

Coarticulation. The theory that sounds are blended together during speech production.

Cognates. Two sounds that differ only in voicing; for example, [p] and [b] are cognates.

Complementary distribution. Sounds that never occur in the same phonetic environment; for example, English [h] and [ŋ] are in complementary distribution.

Consonant. A sound made with marked constriction somewhere along the vocal tract.

Consonant cluster. Two or more consonants occurring within the same syllable in which the sequence of consonants is uninterrupted by vowels.

Continuants. Sounds that can be sustained for extended periods of time. The American English continuant sound classes are fricatives, nasals, liquids, glides, vowels, and diphthongs.

Cooing. A prespeech vocalization containing consonants and vowels produced at the back of the mouth.

CV. Consonant-vowel.

CVC. Consonant-vowel-consonant.

Dark [l]. [l] produced in the velar area. Also called velarized [l].

Deletion. Failure to produce a sound; for example, the pronunciation of "deep" as [di].

Denasalization. An error pattern in which nasal consonants are pronounced as oral consonants (typically oral stops); for example, "me" is pronounced "bi."

Dental. Consonants produced with the tongue tip against the back of the upper front teeth. In American English, alveolar consonants typically are dentalized when they occur prior to an interdental consonant, as in "tenth."

Dentalized. See **Dental.**

Devoicing. Production with partial voicing or complete lack of voicing of sounds that are typically produced with voicing.

Diacritics. Modifications made to phonetic symbols to describe phonetic details; for example, a small raised [ʰ] is a diacritic used to indicate aspiration.

Dialect. A variation of speech caused by the influence of region, social class, or ethnic or racial identification.

Digraph. The name for the sound transcribed [æ].

Diphthong. A sequence of two vowels in which only one is syllabic. The American English diphthongs are [eɪ], [aɪ], [aʊ], [ɔɪ], and [oʊ].

Discrimination training. See **Perception Training.**

Distinctive features. Attributes of sounds that distinguish one sound from another.

Distortion. An inaccurately produced sound.

Dysarthria. Motor speech disorders arising from impairments originating in the peripheral or central nervous system.

Environments. See **Phonetic environments.**

Epenthesis (ePENthesis). An error pattern in which a vowel is inserted between consonants in a consonant cluster; for example, "treat" is pronounced [tərit].

Epsilon. The name for the sound transcribed [ɛ].

Eggressive. The outward flow of air from the mouth or nose.

Final consonant deletion. An error pattern in which a consonant occurring at the end of a syllable or word is deleted; for example, "beet" is pronounced [bi].

Final consonant devoicing. An error pattern in which voiced obstruents are devoiced at the end of a syllable or word; for example, "mead" is pronounced as [mit].

Fricative. A consonant produced with a sufficiently small distance between the articulators to cause a "hissing sound." The American English fricatives are [f], [v], [θ],[ð], [s], [z], [ʃ], and [ʒ].

Front vowels and diphthongs. Vowels in which the tongue tip is the major articulator; the American English front vowels and diphthongs are [i], [ɪ], [eɪ], [ɛ], [æ], [a], [aɪ], and [aʊ].

Frontal lisp. See **Lisping.**

Fronting. An error pattern in which velar consonants (and sometimes postalveolar affricates) are pronounced as alveolar consonants; for example, "key" is pronounced [ti].

Glide. Consonants produced with relatively little constriction between articulators. The American English glides are [j] and [w].

Gliding. An error pattern in which a liquid consonant is pronounced as a glide; for example, "Lee" is pronounced [wi] or (less typically) [ji].

Glottal. Sounds produced at the vocal folds; for example, [h] is a glottal glide.

Glottal replacement. An error pattern in which a consonant is pronounced as a glottal stop; for example, "boot" is pronounced [buʔ].

High vowels. Vowels produced with the tongue raised toward the roof of the mouth. The American English high vowels are [i], [ɪ], [u], and [ʊ].

Homorganic. Sounds produced at the same place of production; for example, in American English [b], [p], [m], and [w] are homorganic.

Homonyms. Words that sound alike but have different meanings; for example, "reed" and the present tense of "read" are homonyms.

Horseshoe. The name for the sound transcribed [ʊ].

Humped [r] and [ɚ]. Production of [r] and [ɚ] with the tongue tip lowered and the bulk of the tongue raised. See **Retroflex [r] and [ɚ]**.

Independent analysis. A type of analysis in which a client's speech abilities are described without reference to the language of the client's community; for example, an independent analysis might describe a client's speech as containing [p b t d], but would not indicate if these consonants are produced correctly relative to the adult language (Stoel-Gammon & Dunn, 1985). Also see **Relational analysis.**

Ingressive. Sounds made with the inward movement of air.

Initial consonant deletion. An error pattern in which the consonant beginning a word is deleted; for example, "bee" is pronounced [i].

Initial sound. A sound beginning a word or syllable.

Interdental. Consonants produced with the tongue tip protruding between the upper and lower front teeth. The American English interdental consonants are [θ] and [ð].

Intervocalic. Consonants occurring between vowels; for example, the second [b] in "baby" is intervocalic. Also see **Syllable position.**

Intonation. See **Prosody.**

Jargon. Sentence-like units in which the sounds are pronounced with little phonetic accuracy. Clients who produce jargon are sometimes said to "know the tune before the words."

Labial. Bilabial and labiodental consonants. The American English labial consonants are [p], [b], [m], [w], [f], and [v].

Labial assimilation. An error pattern in which consonants assimilate to the place of production of a labial consonant; for example, "bead" is pronounced [bib].

Labialization. Pronunciation of consonants with greater-than-expected lip rounding.

Labiodental. Consonants produced with the upper lip and lower teeth. The American English labiodental consonants are [f] and [v].

Lateral. Sounds produced with air flowing over the sides of the tongue. The American English lateral is [l].

Lateral lisp. See **Lisping.**

Lateral [s]. [s] produced with air flowing over the sides of the tongue. The symbol for lateral [s] is [ɬ].

Lateralization. An error pattern in which sounds typically produced with central air emission (most commonly [s] and [z]) are pronounced with lateral air emission; for example, "see" is pronounced [ɬi] (see Appendix 1A for diacritics).

Lip rounding. See **Rounding.**

Lips spread. See **Spreading.**

Light [l]. [l] made at the alveolar place of production. Light [l] typically occurs in syllable-initial position in American English.

Liquid. A class of sounds made with a relatively large aperture between the tongue and the roof of the mouth. The American English liquids are [l] and [r].

Lisping. An error pattern in which alveolar consonants (typically fricatives) are pronounced with the tongue either on or between the front teeth; for example, "see" is pronounced [si]. Also called a frontal lisp. Lateral lisps are the same as lisping except the airflow comes over the sides of the tongue.

Long "s" (pronounced [ɛs]). The name for the sound transcribed [ʃ].

Manner of production. The degree of narrowing in the vocal tract and direction of air flow that occurs during the production of sounds. The American English manner of production classes are stops (oral and nasal), affricates, fricatives, liquids, glides, vowels, and diphthongs.

Maximal pair. See **Word pair.**

Medial sound. See **Word-medial position.**

Metalinguistics. The ability to reflect on language.

Metathesis (MeTAthesis). An error pattern in which the order of sounds in a word is reversed; for example, "peek" is pronounced [kip].

Minimal pair. See **Word pair.**

Multisyllabic. More than one syllable.

Narrow transcription. Transcription containing diacritics to indicate the actual speech sounds produced by a speaker. Narrow transcriptions are enclosed in brackets. See also **Brackets.**

Nasals. A class of consonants made with a lowered velum. The American English nasal stops are [m], [n], and [ŋ]. See also **Nasal stop.**

Nasal stop. A consonant made with the velum lowered and complete closure somewhere in the oral tract.

Nasality. Production of a sound with the velum lowered.

Nasalization. Non-nasal consonants (usually oral stops) are pronounced as nasal stops.

Neutral vowels. Vowels that "stand-in" for many other vowels and diphthongs in unstressed syllables; for example, [ə], [ɪ], and [ʊ] are neutral vowels for many American English speakers.

Noncontrastive. See **Complementary distribution.**

Nonreduplicated babbling. Babbling in which consonants and vowels vary within syllables; for example, "ba-di-du" or "mu-mi." See also **Reduplicated babbling.**

Obstruent. Oral stops, affricates, and fricatives.

Omission. See **Deletion**.

Onset. A linguistic unit theorized by some researchers to occur at the beginning of syllables; for example, [sp] in "spy" and [t] in "toe" are considered onsets in some linguistic theories of syllable structure.

Open. Vowels and diphthongs produced with the tongue lying relatively flat on the floor of the mouth. Open replaces low in the revised International Phonetic Alphabet (International Clinical Phonetics and Linguistic Association, 1992). The American English open vowels and diphthongs are [a], [ɑ], [aɪ], and [aʊ].

Open-mid. Vowels and diphthongs produced with the tongue raised slightly from the floor of the mouth. The category of open-mid replaces mid in the revised International Phonetic Alphabet (International Clinical Phonetics and Linguistic Association, 1992). The American English open-mid vowels and diphthongs are [ɛ], [ʌ], [ɔɪ], and [ɔ].

Open "o" (pronounced [oʊ]). The name for the sound transcribed [ɔ].

Open syllable. Syllable ending with a vowel or diphthong; for example, "bay" and "toe" have open syllables.

Oral stop. Stop consonants that are produced with a raised velum. The American English oral stops are [p], [b], [t], [d], [k], and [g].

Palatal. Place of production at which the tongue approximates the hard palate. The American English palatal consonant is [j].

Perception training. Clinical philosophy that training helps to improve a client's ability to distinguish between different sounds, syllables, and words.

Pharyngeal fricative. A fricative produced in the pharyngeal region. Pharyngeal fricatives sometimes occur in the speech of clients with repaired cleft palates.

Phone. A sound of a language. Every consonant, vowel, and diphthong is a phone.

Phoneme. A sound that is capable of distinguishing between words; for example, [p] and [b] are American English phonemes as illustrated by the words "bee" and "pea."

Phonetic environments. Positions in syllables in which sounds occur; for example, [t] in "beet" occurs in the syllable-final position and [d] in "buddy" occurs in the intervocalic position.

Phonemic transcription. Transcription of the phonemes of a language.

Phonetic transcription. Transcription of the sounds of a language.

Phonetics. The study of the acoustic, psychoacoustic, and production aspects of speech.

Phonological error. A speech error resulting from absent or limited knowledge of the phonological system of the language.

Phonological knowledge. A person's knowledge of the phonological organization of his or her language.

Phonological patterns. See **Phonological processes.**

Phonological processes. Descriptions of systematic differences between the client's speech and the speech of adults in the client's community. Phonological processes are sometimes called phonological patterns.

Phonological rule. A description of the systematic relationship between units in a phonological system.

Phonology. The study of the linguistic organization of sound.

Phonotactics. The rules for the sequential arrangement of speech sounds; for example, an English phonotactic rule is that [sp] is an acceptable word-initial consonant cluster but [ps] is not.

Place of production. The point in the vocal tract at which maximum constriction occurs during production of a sound. Place of production is sometimes called place of articulation.

Postalveolar. A place of production immediately posterior to the alveolar ridge. Postalveolar replaces alveopalatal in the revised edition of the International Phonetic Alphabet (International Clinical Phonetics and Linguistic Association, 1992). The American English postalveolar consonants are [tʃ], [dʒ], [ʃ], and [ʒ].

Postvocalic. Consonants occurring after a vowel in the same syllable; for example, [t] in "eat" [it].

Prevocalic Voicing. An error pattern in which consonants are voiced when they occur before a vowel; for example, "pea" pronounced as [bi].

Primary stress. The major stress in a word; for example, the syllable "tween" carries the primary stress in "between."

Print "a" (pronounced [eɪ]). The name for the sound transcribed [a].

Progressive assimilation. Assimilation due to the influence of an earlier occurring sound on a later occurring sound; for example, [r] is often pronounced with rounded lips in "shriek" because of the lip rounding that occurs in [ʃ]. Also see **Regressive assimilation.**

Prosody. Modifications in pitch, stress, and duration of sounds as they occur in phrases and sentences.

Pure vowel. A vowel that remains relatively unchanged throughout its production; the American English pure vowels are [i], [ɪ], [æ], [a], [ɑ], [ə], [ʌ], [ɔ], [ʊ], and [u].

R-colored vowel. See **Rhotic vowel.**

Reduplicated babbling. Babbling in which syllables are repeated; for example, "ba-ba-ba" or "da-da." Also see **Nonreduplicated babbling.**

Reduplication. An error pattern in which a syllable is repeated; for example, the pronunciation of "water" as [wɑwɑ].

Regressive assimilation. Assimilation resulting from the effect of a later occurring sound on an earlier occurring sound; for example, [n] in "tenth" is often produced as a dental consonant because of the influence of interdental [θ]. See also **Progressive assimilation.**

Relational analysis. Analysis that compares the client's speech to the speech of the client's community (Stoel-Gammon & Dunn, 1985). An example of a relational analysis is the statement, "The client produced [k] as [t]." Also see **Independent analysis.**

Resyllabification. Movement of a sound from its original syllable; for example, [t] in the phrase "It is" often is resyllabified to "I tis" in casual speech.

Retroflex [r] and [ɚ]. [r] and [ɚ] are produced in one of two ways: humped or retroflexed. Retroflex [r] and [ɚ] are produced with the tongue body slightly retracted, the tongue tip raised, and the sides of the back of the tongue against the inside of the teeth. See also **Humped [r] and [ɚ].**

Rhotic vowel. Production of a schwa with an [r]-coloring; for example, the vowel in "merge" and the vowels in "murder."

Rime (also called Rhyme). A linguistic unit within a syllable theorized to include the vowel and any final consonants; for example, the vowel + [nt] in "bent" is considered a rime in some linguistic theories of syllable structure.

Rounding. Lip puckering that accompanies [w] and some back vowels and diphthongs. For many speakers some lip rounding also accompanies [ʃ]. The American English back unrounded vowels are [ʊ], [ʌ], and [ɑ] and the American English back rounded vowels are [u], [oʊ], [ɔ], and [ɔɪ].

S. Syllable.

Schwa. The name for the sound transcribed as [ə].

Semivowels. A consonant that can "stand-in" for a vowel. The American English semivowels are [j] and [w].

Sibilant. Alveolar and postalveolar fricatives and the fricative portion of alveolar and postalveolar affricates.

Singleton. A sound not in a consonant cluster.

Slashes. Transcriptions enclosed by slashes indicate that the sounds are phonemes of the language; for example, /p/ is a phoneme of English. See **Phoneme.**

Sonorants. Sounds produced with relatively unobstructed airflow. The American English sonorant sound classes are nasals, liquids, glides, and vowels.

Spreading. A smile-like stretch of the lips that accompanies [s] and [z] and American English front vowels and diphthongs.

Stimulability. The ability to imitate a sound.

Stop. A class of consonants made with complete closure at some point in the vocal tract. The American English oral stops are [p], [b], [t], [d], [k], and [g] and the American English nasal stops are [m], [n], and [ŋ].

Stopping. An error pattern in which a sound (typically a fricative or affricate) is pronounced as an oral stop; for example, the pronunciation of "see" as [ti].

Stridency deletion. Deletion of strident consonants. See **Strident.**

Strident. Sounds characterized by noisiness resulting from a fast rate of air flow. The English strident consonants are fricatives and affricates in labiodental [f v], alveolar [s z], and postalveolar [tʃ dʒ ʃ ʒ] places of production.

Substitution. Replacement of one sound with another; for example, a substitution of [s] for [t] results in "see" being said as "tee."

Syllable initial position. The beginning of a syllable; for example, [b] in "bug," [sp] in "spy," and [t] in "captain" occur in syllable initial position.

Syllable final position. The end of a syllable; for example, [t] in "pit," [nt] in "mint," and [n] in "captain" occur in syllable final position.

Syllable deletion. An error pattern in which an unstressed syllable is deleted; for example, "banana" is pronounced as [nænə].

Theta. The name for the sound transcribed [θ].

Thorn. The name for the sound transcribed [ɚ].

Unaspirated. Production of a typically aspirated oral stop without aspiration; for example, the pronunciation of "pea" [pʰi] as [pºi].

V. Vowel.

Variegated babbling. See **Nonreduplicated babbling.**

Velar. Place of production made by raising the back of the tongue toward the soft palate. The American English velar consonants are [k], [g], and [ŋ]. Vowels and diphthongs are also made in the velar position, but these are typically called back vowels and back diphthongs rather than velar vowels and velar diphthongs.

Velar assimilation. An error pattern in which consonants assimilate to the place of production of a velar consonant; for example, "teak" is pronounced [kik].

Velarized [l]. See **Dark [l].**

Vocalization. An error pattern in which a syllabic consonant is replaced by a neutral vowel; for example, "beetle" is pronounced [biʔʊ].

Voiced. Sound made with vocal fold vibration.

Voiceless. Sound made without vocal fold vibration.

Voicing. Vibration of the vocal folds.

Vowel. A sound made without marked constriction in the vocal tract.

Vowel neutralization. An error pattern in which a vowel is replaced with a neutral vowel; for example, "bat" is pronounced [bət].

Word-final position. Sounds ending a word; for example, [t] in "boat" is in word-final position. Sounds occurring in word-final position are also said to occur word finally.

Word-initial position. Sounds beginning a word; for example, [p] in "pit" is in word-initial position. Sounds occurring in word-initial position are also said to occur word initially.

Word-medial position. Sounds in the middle of a word; for example, [n] in "final" and [d] in "window" are in word-medial position. Sounds occurring in word-medial position are also said to occur word medially.

Word pairs. Words that differ by a single sound; for example, "pea" and "bee" are word pairs. Word pairs that differ by one distinctive feature in one sound are called minimal pairs (e.g., [p] and [b] in "pea" and "bee"). Word pairs that differ by more than one distinctive feature in one sound are called maximal pairs (e.g., [p] and [m] in "pea" and "me").

APPENDIX 1A
Non-English Symbols and Diacritics

A. Place of Production

Symbol		Description	Examples
[Φ]	[β]**	Bilabial fricatives (two lips approximate each other)	Φ
[̼]		Labiodental oral and nasal stops (upper teeth to lower lip)	p̼ b̼ m̼
[͆]		Dentolabial plosives and nasal (lower teeth to upper lip)	p͆ b͆ m͆
[̪]		Interdentalized (also called lisped) (tongue tip/blade between teeth)	t̪ θ̪ l̪
[̼͆]		Bidental (teeth approximated)	h̼͆ u̼͆
[̼̼͆͆]		Bidental percussive (teeth brought percussively together)	t̼̼͆͆ d̼̼͆͆
	[ɲ]	Palatal nasal (nasal stop made at palatal region)	
[x]	[ɣ]	Velar fricatives (fricatives produced in the velar region)	x ɣ
[fŋ]		Velopharyngeal fricative (fricative made in velopharyngeal region)	fŋ
[ʔ]		Glottal stop (stop produced at vocal folds)	ʔ

B. Manner of Production

Symbol	Description	Examples
[͍]	Labial spreading (lips spread)	s͍ t͍
[̲]	Unrounded (lips at rest, unpursed)	w̲
[̽]	Denasal (little air through nose)	m̽ n̽
[̽]	Nasal escape (air through nose)	p̽ s̽

[̪]	Bladed (produced with tongue blade)	s̪ z̪
[r̮]	[w]-coloring ([r] with a [w]-like quality)	r̮
[ɾ]	Flap (quick stop-like consonant as in "butter")	ɾ
[ˡs]	Lateralized [s] and [z], respectively (air over the sides of tongue)	[ˡs] [ˡz]
[ˮ]	Stronger production (produced with greater force than is typical)	fˮ
[ʔ]	Weaker production (produced with less force than is typical)	m
[↑]	Whistled (high pitched sound)	s↑
[t̥]	Wet sound (produced with excess saliva)	t̥

C. Airstream

[↓]	Ingressive (air moves inward)	p↓
[(X)]	Silent or 'mouthing' (no sound produced)	(s)

D. Vocal Fold Activity

[ᵥ] [ᵥ]	Pre- and post-voicing of sounds (voicing begins or ends later than expected)	ᵥb zᵥ
[₍ₒ₎]	Partial devoicing (normally voiced sound is partially devoiced)	z₍ₒ₎
[₍ᵥ₎]	Partial voicing (normally voiceless sound is partially voiced)	f₍ᵥ₎
[ʰ]	Pre-aspiration (sound begins with aspiration)	ʰp

[°]   Unaspirated   pᵒ tᵒ kᵒ
        (normally aspirated voiceless stops
        produced without aspiration)

E. Syllables and Stress

[̩]   Syllabic   ļ
        (consonant standing as a syllable)

[.]   Syllable boundary   bi.twin
        (separation between syllables)

[´]   Primary stress   bitwín
        (syllable with main stress)

Adapted from: "Recommended phonetic symbols: Extensions of the IPA" by the International Clinical Phonetics and Linguistics Association, (1992), *Clinical Linguistics and Phonetics, 6,* 259–261. With permission.

** = Whenever two symbols are presented, the first is unvoiced and the second is voiced.

CHAPTER

2

Screening and Assessment

The following topics are discussed in this chapter:

Appendix 2C:	Word Probes for Error Patterns
Appendix 2D:	Multiple Error Patterns
Appendix 2E:	Sample Transcription Sheet
Appendix 2F:	Sample Oral Cavity Assessment Form

I. OVERVIEW OF SCREENING

A screening is performed to determine if the client's articulation and phonological development is appropriate for his or her chronological age or developmental age (see Chapter 3, Section VI). Screenings are most successful in settings in which the clients do not show a high incidence of articulation and phonological problems, including well baby clinics, preschools, and grade schools. In settings in which potential clients may have a higher incidence of articulation and phonological disorders (e.g., early intervention programs and Head Start centers), screenings should be undertaken with more caution, because they impose an additional time burden on the clinical staff, who may need to both screen and perform complete assessments on large numbers of clients. Approximately 5 minutes should be allotted for an articulation and phonological screening.

II. NONSTANDARDIZED SCREENINGS

Screenings can be performed using either nonstandardized or published screening instruments. The following is an example of a nonstandardized clinical screening procedure for clients of different chronological ages.

The Setting

Provide screenings (and complete evaluations) in a room sufficiently quiet to hear speech. The room should be clean and free of distractions but not sterile. Toys and other playthings should be kept out of the sight and reach of younger clients. If possible, have parents or professional caregivers familiar with the client present with infants and toddlers. If a client has physical limita-

---

tions or special motoric needs, positioning should be undertaken with guidance from occupational or physical therapy
(Bleile, in press; Bleile & Miller, 1994). If the client has a medical
condition, a nurse or other qualified staff member knowledgeable about the client's medical status should be consulted to rule
out the existence of medical complications that would either
interfere with the assessment or exacerbate the client's medical
problems (Bleile & Miller, in press).

A. All Ages

If a caregiver is present, ask if he or she is concerned about the
client's speech. Spend a moment to study the client's face, looking
for signs of gross structural abnormalities. If time permits and the
client is cooperative, open the client's mouth and shine a penlight
at the roof of the mouth to look for repaired or submucous clefts.
The latter often appear as a blue tint at midline. With infants it
often is easier to insert a gloved finger in the mouth than to peer in
with a penlight. Be sure to wash any powder off the glove before
inserting it in the client's mouth. Note any gross abnormalities in
teeth (including malocclusions) and tongue size. Ask the client's
caregivers questions to determine if risk factors are present (see
Section VII), which might suggest that the client should receive a
full evaluation, even if a delay in articulation and phonological
development does not yet exist.

B. Infants (9 to 12 Months)

Ask the caregiver to help elicit vocalizations. Also ask, "Does your
baby make babbling noises?" If the caregiver answers yes, probe
further by asking, "What do the sounds sound like?" The purpose
of these questions is to determine if the child engages in reduplicated babbling (repetition of identical consonants, such as "ba
ba") or nonreduplicated babbling (repetition of different consonants, such as "ba da"), skills that emerge between 7 and 9 months
of age. Refer the infant for a speech-language evaluation if the
caregiver indicates that the child does not make noise or does not
engage in reduplicated or nonreduplicated babbling.

C. Toddlers (18 to 24 Months)

Ask the caregiver to play with the child to elicit speech. Also ask the caregiver: "Does your child speak yet?" or "Does your child use words to communicate?" The purpose of this question is to discover if the child speaks more than three words, a skill that emerges near 13 months of age. If the caregiver answers affirmatively, ask "What words does your child say — can you give me examples?" If the caregiver answers any of these questions negatively, refer the child for a speech-language evaluation.

D. Preschoolers, School-age Children, and Adults

Ask the client, "What did you have for breakfast today?" or "What did you do today?" Also compare the client's development to age norms on consonant and consonant cluster acquisition using an instrument of the clinician's choosing or the one provided in Appendix 2A. If the client fails to produce the consonants and consonant clusters expected of persons of his or her age, a referral should be made for a complete speech-language evaluation.

III. Published Screening Instruments

If the decision is made to use a published screening instrument, the clinician has a wide range of instruments from which to choose. The most widely used instruments are listed below.

Predictive Screening Test of Articulation (PSTA)

Authors: Van Riper, C. & Erickson, J. (1968). Predictive screening test of articulation. *Journal of Speech and Hearing Disorders,* 34, 214–219.

Comments: Developed to identify children whose speech is likely to improve without treatment; intended for use with first graders.

Preschool Language Scale 3 (PLS-3)

Authors: Zimmerman, I., Steiner, V., & Pond, R. (1992). *Preschool language scale 3.* . Columbus, OH: Charles E. Merrill.

Comments: A language test that contains a screening subtest for speech; intended for use with children 1 through 7 years.

Quick Screen of Phonology (Quick Screen or QSP)

Authors: Bankson, N., & Bernthal, J. (1990). *Quick screen of phonology.* Chicago: Riverside Press.

Comments: A relatively new picture naming test developed by two highly regarded clinical investigators; intended for use with children 3 through 7 years old.

Screening Deep Test of Articulation (Screening Deep Test)

Author: McDonald, E. (1968). *Screening Deep Test of Articulation.* Pittsburgh: Stanwix House.

Comments: Offers a relatively in-depth screening (90 items); intended for use with children kindergarten through 3rd grade.

Speech and Language Screening Test for Preschool Children (Fluharty)

Author: Fluharty, N. (1978). *Speech and Language Screening Test for Preschool Children.* Bingingham, MS: Teaching Resources.

Comments: Elicits speech using real objects; intended for use with children 2 through 6 years old.

Templin-Darley Screening Test

Authors: Templin, M., & Darley, F. (1969). *Templin-Darley Screening Test.* Iowa City: University of Iowa Bureau of Education Research and Service.

Comments: A well-known screening test; intended for use with children 3 through 8 years old.

Test of Minimal Articulation Competence (T-MAC)

Author: Secord, W. (1981). *Test of Minimal Articulation Competence.* San Antonio: The Psychological Corporation.

Comments: A complete assessment instrument that includes a quick (3 to 5 minute) screening test.

IV. OVERVIEW OF ARTICULATION AND PHONOLOGICAL ASSESSMENTS

A complete articulation and phonological assessment is performed to achieve one or more of three goals:

To determine the client's current level of and prognosis for future articulation and phonological development,

To determine if the client's problem is severe enough to warrant intervention, and

To provide information useful in planning treatment, if that is found to be warranted.

A. Steps in Articulation and Phonological Assessment

Typically, a complete articulation and phonological assessment is part of a speech-language evaluation. The articulation and phonological assessment consists of three sections: initial observation, collection of the speech sample, and hypothesis testing.

1. **Initial Observation.** During the initial observation the clinician listens to the client's spontaneous speech, makes notes about particular speech errors, and formulates an initial impression of the client's perceived intelligibility. Depending on the client's developmental level, the spontaneous speech sample can be obtained by asking the client to describe a picture, to respond to questions such as "What did you have for breakfast?" or simply by listening to the client speak during conversation. Approximately 3 to 5 minutes are allotted for the initial observation.

2. **Collection of the Speech Sample.** The clinician collects a speech sample for later analysis using either nonstandardized procedures, published instruments, or a combination of both. The relative strengths and limitations of nonstandardized procedures and published instruments are listed in Tables 2–1 and 2–2, respectively. As summarized in Table 2–3, nonstandardized assessments are often the primary or sole form of assessment for clients in Stage 1 or Stage 2, are used in conjunction with standardized assessment instruments for clients in Stage 3, and may serve as an adjunct to standardized tests for clients in Stage 4. Whatever combination of nonstandardized and standardized assessments are performed, the clinician should allow 10 to 30 minutes for collection of the speech sample, depending on the extent of the client's articulation and phonological problems.

Table 2-1. Strengths and limitations of nonstandardized assessment procedures.

Variable	Characteristics
Strengths	Flexible procedures allow the clinician to adapt the assessment to the client's learning style
	Can be used with clients who are not testable by other means
	Can be used when no published test is suitable to the client's needs or developmental level
	Often provides more in-depth analysis than typically is provided by a published assessment instrument
Limitations	Requires greater knowledge by the clinician
	Use of flexible procedures may impair reliability
	Some nonstandardized procedures require more time than is available in most clinical settings

Table 2-2. Strengths and limitations of standardized assessment instruments.

Variable	Characteristics
Strengths	Promotes reliability by use of standardized procedures and speech samples
	Provides an overview of important speech assessment topics
	Often is time-efficient
	Results are often accepted by insurance companies and other third party payers
Limitations	Not all clients have sufficient cognitive and attention skills to perform well on published tests
	Many published instruments do not analyze speech in sufficient depth to be used with clients who have severe articulation and phonological disorders

Table 2–3. Use of non-standardized procedures and standardized instruments at four developmental levels.

Developmental Level	Assessment Strategy
Stage 1	Primarily nonstandardized assessments supplemented by standardized instruments
Stage 2	Primarily nonstandardized assessments supplemented by standardized instruments
Stage 3	Combination of nonstandardized procedures and standardized instruments
Stage 4	Primarily standardized assessment instruments supplemented by nonstandardized assessment procedures

3. **Hypothesis Testing.** Hypothesis testing is undertaken to obtain additional information about the client's articulation and phonological disorder. During the collection of the speech sample, for example, a client might pronounce "key" as [ti], raising the question of whether this pronunciation results from an error pattern that turns all velar stops into alveolar stops. Alternately, the client might produce [f] correctly in one word, and the clinician may want to know if the client is able to produce [f] correctly in other words. In general, hypothesis testing requires from between a few minutes to 30 minutes, depending on the nature and complexity of the client's articulation and phonological problems. Time permitting, hypothesis testing is undertaken during the evaluation session at which the speech sample is collected. Hypothesis testing may also be undertaken over several sessions concurrent with the onset of treatment.

Hypothesis testing can be undertaken using a wide variety of procedures. The author's preference is to use word probes such as those provided in Appendixes 2B and 2C. These probes can be used either to test individual sounds (sound probes) or error patterns (error probes). Word probes also provide a time efficient means to perform pre-tests and post-tests and to search for key phonetic environments and key words (see Section V in Chapter 3). Typically, word probes are not used to test all the client's errors, but focus instead on the sounds and error patterns that seem likely treatment goals. To illustrate, a client's speech might show the error patterns of Fronting, Stopping, Prevocalic Voicing, and deletion of abutting consonants word medially (e.g., the pronunciation of "window" as "widow."). In this situation, it would be appropriate to perform word probes to test hypotheses related to Fronting, Stopping, and Prevocalic Voicing, but not the error pattern affecting abutting consonants word medially. This is because, given the nature of the client's other error patterns, the error pattern affecting medial consonants is not likely to be selected as an early treatment goal.

What's in a Name

Error patterns include all errors that affect more than one sound. This includes such traditional articulation categories as lisping and lateralization, as well as what are called phonological processes or phonological patterns. The term error pattern was chosen to avoid biasing the discussion to either an articulation or phonological perspective.

V. NONSTANDARDIZED ASSESSMENTS

The following are procedural guidelines for undertaking a nonstandardized assessment.

Multiple Error Patterns

Most clients in Stage 2 and Stage 3 experience difficulties with more than one aspect of articulation and phonological development. A client, for example, may experience problems with both pronouncing fricatives and producing voiceless consonants. The result may be two error patterns: Stopping and Prevocalic Voicing, both of which may occur in the same word. A client, for example, might say "see" as [di] because the com-
(continued)

bination of Stopping and Prevocalic Voicing converts [s] into [d]. Identifying the effects of multiple error patterns can be challenging. The information in Appendix 2D illustrates how commonly occurring combinations of error patterns may affect consonants and consonant clusters.

A. Sample Size

In general, a nonstandardized assessment requires a sample of between 50 to 100 utterances. Smaller samples are typically collected during initial evaluations with clients in Stage 1 and Stage 2, because these clients often vocalize and speak less. Whenever possible, two or three productions of the same words should be obtained for clients in Stage 2 and early Stage 3, because these clients are often variable in how they say words (see the discussion of short-term goals in Chapter 4).

B. Transcription System

Speech is transcribed using the International Phonetic Alphabet (IPA) or an equivalent system. As summarized in Table 2-4, the client's level of articulation and phonological development largely determines whether whole words or isolated sounds are transcribed. With clients in Stage 1, either the entire vocalization is transcribed phonetically or a checklist system is used (see Appendix 3J). Whole words are transcribed when the client is in Stage 2 or Stage 3, because the presence of a sound in one part of a word can affect the production of another sound elsewhere in the word. Typically, isolated sounds are transcribed if the client is in Stage 4.

Table 2-4. Transcription at four levels of development.

Developmental Level	Type of Transcription
Stage 1	Entire vocalization or checklist
Stage 2	Whole word
Stage 3	Whole word
Stage 4	Individual sounds or check mark system

The Reluctant Child

If a young child appears reluctant to enter the evaluation room, ask "Do you like to play?" Most children nod or say yes and then come willingly. Another technique that sometimes works is to tell the child that you have a new toy you want the child to play with, which is a very special toy that the child will be the first one to use.

C. Non-English Symbols and Diacritics

Different non-English symbols and diacritics are likely to be needed depending on the client's level of articulation and phonological development. (See Appendix 1A for the list of non-English symbols and diacritics used in this book.)

1. **Stage 1.** Stage 1 vocalizations are not well-described by most systems of non-English symbols and diacritics. For most clinical purposes, a checklist system bypasses the need for diacritics (Vannucci, 1994). Appendix 3J contains a sample vocalization checklist. If detailed phonetic transcriptions are needed, the reader is referred to discussions in Oller (1992), Proctor (1989), and Stark (1980).

2. **Stage 2.** The **non-English symbols and diacritics** most likely to be needed for transcription of the speech of clients in Stage 2 include labiodental stops (often produced for bilabial stops), bilabial fricatives (often produced for [f] and [v]), unaspirated voiceless stops (often produced in place of aspirated stops), wet sounds (wet sounding speech often occurs in clients with oral motor problems), and glottal stops. The most difficult of these sounds to hear are unaspirated, voiceless stops and glottal stops.

   a. **Labiodental Stops.** Labiodental stops often sound like bilabial stops, but can be identified by the upper teeth touching the lower lip, which may be similar or identical to the position used for [f] and [v].

Diacritics

Extensive use of diacritics is time consuming and leads to transcriptions in which the phonetic symbols become lost among all the accompanying wiggles, wavy lines, and circles. On the other hand, using too few diacritics results in missing clinically significant aspects of speech. The following general rules may prove helpful in deciding which diacritics to include in transcriptions:

• Include only those diacritics that are clinically relevant. Do not attempt the nearly impossible task of transcribing all the phonetic details of the client's speech.
• On the top of the first page of the transcription sheet list the diacritics you are likely to need based on the client's level of articulation and phonological development, recognizing that all of them might not be needed or that other diacritics may also be needed.
• While transcribing the client's speech, if you hear the client produce a sound in a way that you cannot readily describe, transcribe the closest approximation of the sound you are able to make, and place an "X" under it. For example, if you hear something "[s]-like," but somehow different than standard [s], transcribe it as [s] with an "X" underneath. Continue placing "X" under the [s] until you are able to identify how the client is producing the sound. When this occurs, define the "X." For example, you might indicate at the bottom of the page that "X = voiceless lateral postalveolar fricative."
• Exclude diacritics that describe relatively minor, predictable aspects of speech production. For example, do not use diacritics to indicate that [s] is produced with lip rounding when preceding [w] in "sweet" or that [r] is usually produced without voicing when following voiceless consonants in such words as "pride."
• Exclude diacritics that describe aspects of speech that the client produces in an adult manner. For example, do not use diacritics to indicate stress patterns and syllable boundaries that conform to that of the adult language. To illustrate, do not use a diacritic to indicate stress if the client says "begin" with stress on the second syllable, but do so if the client says the same word with stress on the first syllable.

b. **Bilabial Fricatives.** Bilabial fricatives often are perceived as sounding like a cross between a fricative and a glide and can be identified by the client's lips coming together close or identical to the position for [p] and [b].

c. **Voiceless, Unaspirated Stops.** Voiceless, unaspirated stops are often mistaken for voiced stops. There are several options to practice hearing these sounds.

   (1) **Perception.** Most American English speakers who hear voiceless unaspirated stops report that the sound "jumps" between the aspirated voiceless sound and its voiced counterpart (e.g., [pʰ] and [b]). If you hear a [b] that "jumps" in perception between [pʰ] and [b], it may be a voiceless unaspirated stop.

   (2) **Phonetic Drills.** Several phonetic drill books have tapes of voiceless, unaspirated stops (Edwards, 1986; Shriberg & Kent, 1982).

   (3) **Native Speaker.** Ask a speaker of a language that has voiceless, unaspirated stops to produce [p], [t], or [k].

   (4) **Production.** Sometimes, making a sound facilitates hearing it better. To do this, place your hand in front of your mouth and say [pʰ]. Feel the puff of air on your hand. Now, keep repeating [pʰ], working to reduce the puff of air on your hand. When the puff of air is gone, but the sound is not quite [b], it is probably a voiceless unaspirated [p].

d. **Glottal Stops.** There are several ways to train yourself to hear glottal stops:

   (1) **Word-initial.** The word "ice," if said forcefully, begins with a strong glottal stop. Repeat the word several times aloud, tuning your ear to the glottal stop.

   (2) **Word-final.** A glottal stop at the end of a word sounds like the preceding vowel was cut off very suddenly. Say "bee" several times, cutting off the vowel each time.

   (3) **Between Vowels.** Glottal stops that replace consonants in the middle of words (as in "funny") sound

like someone trying to imitate a Cockney accent. To practice, try saying "funny" several times with a Cockney accent.

3. **Stage 3.** The same non-English symbols and diacritics are used to transcribe the speech of clients in Stage 2 and Stage 3 (labiodental stops, unaspirated voiceless stops, wet sounds, and glottal stops). Additional diacritics likely to be needed include [w] coloring of [r], as well as lisped, lateralized, and bladed productions of [s] and [z].

   a. **[w] Colored [r].** [w] coloring of [r] often is perceived as being between [w] and [r].

   b. **Lisping.** During lisping [s] and [z] are produced with the client's tongue either touching the teeth or protruding slightly between the teeth as for [θ] or [ð]; however, the tongue may be either more forward or retracted than for [θ] and [ð]. Air may also be released over the sides of the tongue, in which case the sound is called a lateral lisp ([ls] and [lz]).

   c. **Lateralized.** Lateralized [s] and [z] can be identified by feeling for release of air by placing the hand near the sides of the client's mouth.

   d. **Bladed.** Bladed production of [s] and [z] often is perceived as an [s] or [z] with [ʃ]- or [ʒ]-like qualities, although the tongue may not be retracted as far back as it is for [ʃ] and [ʒ].

4. **Stage 4.** Transcriptions for clients in Stage 4 are likely to need the same non-English symbols and diacritics as for clients in Stage 3 ([w] coloring of [r] and lisped, lateralized, and bladed production of [s] and [z]).

D. Information Maintenance

There are no agreed-on methods to maintain client information. The client's utterances can simply be transcribed on a piece of paper or on a sheet such as that presented in Appendix 2E. The use of a form is illustrated in Table 2–5.

Table 2–5. Example of a transcription sheet.

Word	Transcription	Environments			Other Environments		
		#___	V_V	___#	___	___	___
	b						
pea	p̸i	p→b					
	ø̸tuø̸						
stoop	s̸tup̸	st→ø̸t		p→ø̸			

1. **Word.** The word is the presumed meaning of the word (or phrase). A question mark is used if the clinician is uncertain of the client's meaning. If a client points to a dog and says [du], for example, the word is "dog." If the clinician is uncertain if "dog" is the presumed meaning of [du], the word is "?dog."

2. **Transcription.** The transcription is the phonetic rendition of the word (or phrase). The transcription of "pea," for example, is [pi]. Differences between this and the client's pronunciation of the word are indicated directly above the sounds in error. The [b] for [p] pronunciation in "pea," for example, is indicated by transcribing [b] above the crossed out transcription of [p]. Deletion of consonants (as occurs for [s] in "stoop") is indicated by the null (zero) sign.

3. **Environments.** The environments indicate where the sound or sounds occurred. The most commonly used environments are beginnings of words (#___), ends of words (___#), and between vowels (V___V) (see Chapter 1 for definitions of environments). Vowels are usually indicated by "V." If the client pronounces "stoop" as [tu], for example, the first error occurs in a word-initial environment and the second error occurs in a word-final environment.

4. **Other Environments.** Other environments are environments that may be added as need arises. A clinician, for example, might add a syllable-initial environment (S___) to describe the production of [h] in words such as "behind."

E. Recording Speech

Decisions must also be made as to whether video or audio tapes will be used for later transcription and analysis.

1. **Repetitions.** If recording the client's speech, repeat the word after the client so that you can later identify what the client said. Also say in a quiet voice any characteristics that might be difficult to identify on the tape (e.g., "Oh, I saw your tongue between your teeth").

2. **Recording Devices.** Select a high-quality recording device from among the wide variety of excellent recording equipment available commercially.

3. **Microphones.** If possible, record speech samples using a lapel microphone unless the client's movements appear likely to produce too much noise. Free standing microphones are often best to use with these clients. If possible, two microphones are used in case the client moves around.

4. **Recording Procedures.** Shriberg (1993) recommends the following recording procedures:

    a. Record the speech in a quiet environment.

    b. If the environment is noisier than optimal, reduce the mouth-to-microphone distance if the noise is constant, or have the client repeat the utterance if the noise is transient.

    c. Use high-quality recorders with an impedance-matched external microphone and high-quality cassette tapes.

    d. Place the cassette deck on a different surface from the microphone and as far away as possible to avoid noise from the tape deck interfering with the recording.

    e. Place the microphone approximately 6 to 8 inches from the client's lips.

    f. Adjust the volume control so the client's vowels cause the VU meter to peak just below the distortion range (In general, volume levels between one half to two thirds of the highest volume yield the best signal-to-noise ratios).

To Record or Not Record

If you believe recording improves your clinical work, then by all means record, but remember that it takes just as long to listen to an audio tape or watch a video tape as it did to make the recording and that transcribing the tape is likely to require much additional time. Because of the time it takes, extensive recording of clients' speech is probably not practical outside of university settings. For this reason, many clinicians restrict use of recordings to challenging clinical cases, for use for educational purposes, and — less often — to document clinical progress.

F. Types of Speech Samples

One of the most important clinical decisions involves the types of speech samples to collect. Methods for collecting speech samples are listed in Table 2-6.

Table 2-6. Methods used to collect a speech sample.

Elicitation Techniques	Definition
Spontaneous speech	Naturally occurring speech
Elicited speech	
Naming	Single words typically elicited through naming objects or pictures
Sentence completion	Single words typically elicited through the client finishing the clinician's sentence
Delayed Imitation	Single words typically elicited through placing a short phrase between the clinician's model and the client's response
Imitation	Single words typically elicited through the client's immediate imitation of the clinician's model

1. **Spontaneous Speech.** Spontaneous speech is the preferred sampling technique because it is most representative of how the client talks (Ingram, 1994; Morrison & Shriberg, 1992; Morrison & Shriberg, 1994). The major limitation of spontaneous speech samples is the length of time it can take to transcribe them, especially if the client speaks in sentences of three or more words. Further, longer utterances usually must be tape recorded to be transcribed, which adds greatly to the time needed to complete the analysis. For this reason, many clinicians prefer to spend a few minutes early in the session listening to the client's spontaneous speech, perhaps making notes about particular speech errors and the client's level of severity and/or intelligibility. The initial impression of the client's spontaneous speech is then used to guide the subsequent analysis of the client's elicited speech.

2. **Elicited Speech.** There are four major speech elicitation techniques: naming, sentence completion, delayed imitation, and imitation.

   a. **Naming.** Naming involves asking a client to name pictures or objects. For example, the clinician asks, "What is thio?" or ongogoo in an objoot identification gnme in which the client names objects pulled from a shoe box.

   b. **Sentence Completion.** Sentence completion involves asking the client to end a sentence begun by the clinician. For example, the clinician might pick up an object or picture and say, "Here/This is a _____ ." A useful variation of this procedure which tests morphological endings is to say, "Here is a _____ . Here is another _____ . Now I have two _____ ." One advantage of sentence completion tasks over naming procedures is that sentence completion elicits speech somewhat faster. More importantly, sentence completion tasks direct the client to say the words you want to elicit.

   c. **Delayed Imitation.** Delayed imitation involves placing a short phrase between the clinician's request to say a word or phrase and the client's response. For example, the clinician says, "This is a dog." Now you say it./"Now you say it." The phrase provides a small amount of time during which the client must hold the word in memory, which presumably makes this task slightly more reflective of cognitive skills than immediate imitation. Delayed imitation is quick and useful when the clinician wants to elicit a large number of words from the client.

d. **Immediate Imitation.** Immediate imitation involves having the client immediately repeat something said by the clinician. For example, the clinician says, "Say these words after me," followed by the words. Immediate imitation is the least natural elicitation technique, but it has the advantage of offering a speedy way to elicit a large number of words.

H. Elicitation Activities

Activities used to collect speech samples change according to the client's chronological age and for clients who have intellectual impairments or cognitive deficits, level of cognitive development.

Leave Your Dignity at the Door

The curricula of most graduate schools does not include course work on smacking your lips, singing, tickling, and puffing out your cheeks, but these are some of the techniques that often work best with infants. The best advice for working with the youngest of clients is to leave your dignity at the door and enjoy yourself.

---

1. **Infants and Toddlers.** The optimal elicitation technique is to observe the child interact with his or her caregivers. Begin by asking the caregiver, "Will you play with your child a few minutes so I can get a better idea how your child sounds?" If the caregiver is not available, the clinician should interact with the child. Whether the caregiver or clinician is the elicitor, have the following objects present and introduce and remove them one at a time to avoid overwhelming the child.

   a. **0 to 6 Months.** Infants 0 to 6 months old tend to vocalize while shaking a small rattle, listening to a music box start and stop, watching a black and white mobile, holding a hand-held or noise-making toy, and playing with a simple busy box.

The Problem May Not Be Speech

Sometimes a client's articulation and phonological disorder is the first indication of larger problems in language and cognitive development. In some cases, a client's family will say their child has a speech problem, even when they suspect that their child may have more extensive developmental problems, because a speech problem seems correctable and is easier to deal with emotionally. Other times, a client's family will say their child has a speech problem, having no inkling that their child's speech is part of a larger picture of developmental difficulties. Because language and cognitive disorders sometimes manifest first as speech problems, the clinician should perform a thorough language evaluation of all young clients who are referred for problems with speech development.

---

b. **6 to 12 Months.** Infants 6 to 12 months old tend to vocalize while looking in a mirror; watching bubbles; or playing with pop-up toys or manipulable toys, such as, a toy drum and toy cars.

c. **12 to 18 Months.** Toddlers 12 to 18 months old tend to speak while riding a wagon or tricycle, looking at a simple picture book with an adult, putting together and taking apart Mr. and Mrs. Potato Head, or "talking" on a play telephone.

d. **18 to 24 Months.** Toddlers 18 to 24 months old tend to speak while playing with and dressing a doll, looking at a picture book with an adult, playing with building blocks, putting together a big-piece puzzle, or "talking" on a play telephone.

2. **Preschoolers (2 to 4 Years).** The following ideas may help elicit speech either directly or through the help of a caregiver.

a. **Reading.** Read a picture book with the client and have the client name and describe actions in the pictures.

b. **Shopping.** Play "shopping" with pretend food, play money, and a cash register.

c. **Tea Party.** Have a tea party or make a meal using toy dishes, utensils, and cooking equipment.

d. **Dress a Doll.** Help the child dress a doll. The adult holds a doll, and the child names the pieces of clothing to put on the doll. Alternately, the adult wears a puppet, and the child tells the puppet how to dress the doll.

e. **Puppets.** The adult and the child wear finger or hand puppets and have the puppets take turns telling stories such as Little Red Riding Hood or The Three Little Pigs.

f. **Broken Toy.** Present the child with a broken toy with a missing part and ask the child, "What's wrong?" or "Why won't it work?"

g. **Misnaming.** The adult (or a puppet) misnames common objects, saying things like, "This is a dog" while pointing to a toy cat. The hope is that the client will correct the adult by giving the appropriate name for the object.

3. **Late Preschoolers and Younger Grade School Children.** The following ideas help to elicit speech from late preschoolers (4 to 5 years of age) and younger grade school children (through 3rd grade).

a. **Spontaneous Speech**

(1) **Family Photos.** If possible, ask the client's caregivers to bring in a family photo album and have the client tell you about the album photos.

(2) **Picture Sequence Cards.** Lay out picture sequence cards and have the client use the pictures to tell a story.

(3) **Most Favorite/Least Favorite.** Ask the child to tell you what is his or her favorite/least favorite cartoon, television program, food, animal, and so on. Alternately, ask the child, "What did you have for breakfast?" or "Where's your favorite place to go in the entire world?"

(4) **Broken Toy.** Present the child with a broken toy and ask him or her to tell you what is wrong and how to fix it.

(5) **Tell a Story.** Give the child a picture book and ask him or her to tell a story. Alternately, wear finger or hand puppets and either have the child tell a story to the puppet or have the puppet tell the story.

(6) **Play Acting.** Play act with the child using favorite activities and characters, for example, playing house, going grocery shopping, or pretending to be Bugs Bunny, or the Power Rangers.

(7) **Explain a Game.** Have the child explain a game to you or a puppet, for example, jacks, Cootie, Old Maid, or hide-and-seek.

(8) **Funny Clothes.** Enter the room wearing something funny (perhaps upside down toy glasses), hoping the child will notice and discuss it.

(9) **Treasure Hunt.** Play treasure hunt in which the clinician visually impairs a stuffed animal with sunglasses, so that the child has to describe where the treasure is hidden in the room.

(10) **Bizarre Questions.** Ask the child bizarre questions, for example, "Are you married?" or "I like your shoes. Can I have them?"

b. **Single Words**

(1) **Turn Over the Cards.** Play a game in which the child is allowed to turn over and remove picture cards from a table after naming what is on the card.

(2) **Bingo.** Play Bingo, allowing the child to pick a picture from a bag, name the picture, and match it to a sheet in front of him or her.

(3) **Tossing Games.** Play ball or bean bag toss, instructing the child to toss a ball or a bean bag to a board with pictures on it and to name the pictures he or she hits.

(4) Steps. Place picture cards on steps and have the client climb the steps, naming the picture cards on each step.

(5) Toy Car. Place cards on a table or the floor and let the client drive a toy car over the cards, naming each card the car rolls over. Alternately, have the child roll a ball and name the card on which the ball stops.

(6) Magic Box. Show the child a "magic box" or a lunch bag. Play a game in which the child reaches into and pulls out and names objects or pictures from the box or bag. Alternately, draw a picture of a cartoon character with a big mouth on a piece of paper, for example, Cookie Monster or a lion. Place the picture over the opening of a cardboard box and instruct the client to reach in and tell you what is in Cookie Monster's (or the lion's) mouth.

(7) Lights Off. Place objects around the treatment room before the client arrives. When the client arrives, turn off the light and have the client shine a flashlight around the room, naming objects as they are found.

(8) Play Teacher. Let the child play teacher by wearing glasses and using a pointer to name objects placed around the room.

4. **Older Grade School Children and Adolescents.** Ask the client one or more of the following questions.

   a. **Blame.** Have you ever been blamed for something you didn't do?

   b. **Dump Truck.** What would you do if someone dropped a dump truck of popcorn in your living room?

   c. **Ball on a Roof.** Can you tell me how to get a ball off a roof?

   d. **Christmas Tree.** How do you decorate a Christmas tree?

   e. **Sandwich.** Can you tell me how you make a peanut butter and jelly sandwich?

5. **Adults.** Ask the client one or more of the following questions.

    a. **Today.** What were you doing before you came here today?

    b. **Store.** Would you describe the route from your home to the nearest grocery store?

    c. **Kitchen.** Would you describe your kitchen for me?

VI. PUBLISHED ASSESSMENT INSTRUMENTS

The following published instruments offer a wide range of approaches to assess articulation and phonological disorders. Specific procedural guidelines for the tests are included with the individual assessment instruments. When applicable. I indicate whether the test instrument is oriented primarily to analyzing error patterns (typically, phonological processes) or individual sounds (typically, consonants and consonant clusters). Unless otherwise noted, each test requires approximately 30 minutes to complete.

Arizona Articulation Proficiency Scale (Arizona or AAPS)

Authors: Fudala, B., & Reynolds, W. (1986). *Arizona Articulation Proficiency Scale.* Los Angeles: Western Psychological Services.

Comments: A traditional test of individual sounds.

Assessment Link Between Phonology and Articulation (ALPHA)

Author: Lowe, R. (1986). *Assessment Link Between Phonology and Articulation.* East Moline, IL: LinguiSystems.

Comments: A carefully designed assessment instrument for children 3 years and older.

The Assessment of Phonological Processes — Revised (APP-R)

Author: Hodson, B. (1986). *The Assessment of Phonological Processes — Revised.* Danville, IL: The Interstate Publishers and Printers.

Comments: One of the most popular tests of error patterns; intended for children with multiple error patterns; takes about 50 minutes to complete. Also comes in a computer version.

The Assessment of Phonological Processes — Spanish (APP-S)

Author: Hodson, B. (1986). *The Assessment of Phonological Processes — Spanish.* San Diego, CA: Los Amigos Association.

Comments: The Spanish version of the popular APP-R.

Austin Spanish Articulation Test (ASAT)

Author: Carrow, E. (1974). *Austin Spanish Articulation Test*. Austin, TX: Teaching Resources Corporation.

Comments: A traditional test of individual sounds; one of the few tests available to assess Spanish speakers.

Bankson-Bernthal Test of Phonology (Bankson-Bernthal)

Authors: Bankson, N., & Bernthal, J. (1990). *Bankson-Bernthal Test of Phonology*. Chicago: Riverside Press.

Comments: A carefully designed error pattern assessment instrument developed for children 3;0–7;11 by two highly respected clinical investigators.

Children's Speech Intelligibility Test (CSIT)

Authors: Kent, R., Miolo, G., & Bloedel, S. (1994). Children's speech intelligibility test. *American Journal of Speech-Language Pathology, 3,* 81–95.

Comments: A word-recognition test of intelligibility for children with limited speech abilities; this test is in the developmental stage, and the authors do not necessarily recommend it for use in intelligibility assessment

Clinical Probes of Articulation Consistency (C-PAC)

Author: Secord, W. (1981). *Clinical Probes of Articulation Consistency*. San Antonio, TX: The Psychological Corporation.

Comments: A collection of probes for individual consonants and vowels; requires approximately 5 minutes per consonant probe and 10 minutes per vowel probe.

Compton-Hutton Phonological Assessment (Compton-Hutton)

Authors: Compton, A., & Hutton, S. (1978). *Compton-Hutton Phonological Assessment*. San Francisco: Carousel House.

Comments: A test of error patterns that contains a good selection of multisyllabic words; intended for children with multiple error patterns.

Computer Analysis of Phonological Processes: Version 1.0. [Apple II series computer programs]

Author: Hodson, B. (1985). *Computer Analysis of Phonological Processes* Version 1. Danville, IL: Interstate Printers and Publishers.

Comments: Computer version of the popular APP-R.

Computerized Profiling

Authors: Long, S., & Fey, M. (1994). H. *Computerized Profiling*. Austin, TX: Psychological Corporation.

Comments: A new computer analysis for the Macintosh computer program and MS-DOS systems.

A Deep Test of Articulation (McDonald Deep Test)

Author: McDonald, E. (1964). *A Deep Test of Articulation*. Pittsburgh, PA: Stanwix House.

Comments: A test of individual sounds that provides detailed information on phonetic environments; comes in picture and sentence forms; requires approximately 1 hour to complete.

The Edinburgh Articulation Test (Edinburgh)

Authors: Anthony, A., Bogle, D., Ingram, T., & McIsaac, M. (1971). *The Edinburgh Articulation Test*. Edinburgh: E & S Livingston.

Comments: A traditional test of individual sounds and consonant clusters developed for children between 2 years, 6 months to 6 years old.

Fisher-Logemann Test of Articulation Competence (Fisher-Logemann)

Authors: Fisher, H., & Logemann, J. (1971). *Fisher-Logemann Test of Articulation Competence*. Boston, MA: Houghton Mifflin.

Comments: A traditional test of individual sounds.

Goldman-Fristoe Test of Articulation (Goldman-Fristoe or GFTA)

Authors: Goldman, R., & Fristoe, M. (1986). *Goldman-Fristoe Test of Articulation*. Circle Pines, MN: American Guidance Service.

Comments: A well-respected test of individual sounds for late preschoolers and school-age children.

The Khan-Lewis Phonological Analysis (Khan-Lewis or KLPA)

Authors: Khan, L., & Lewis, N. (1986). *The Khan-Lewis Phonological Analysis*. Circle Pines, MN: American Guidance Service.

Comments: A well-designed test that uses pictures from the GFTA to identify error patterns.

Logical International Phonetic Programs (LIPP)

Authors: Oller, K., & Delgado, R. (1990). *Logical International Phonetic Programs*. Miami, FL: Intelligent Hearing Systems.

Comments: Offers in-depth speech analysis for Version 1.03 (MS-DOS computers).

The Macintosh Interactive System for Phonological Analysis

Authors: Masterson, J., & Pagan, F. (1994). *The Macintosh Interactive System for Phonological Analysis*. San Antonio, TX: The Psychological Corporation.

Comments: A new procedure to analyze speech using a Macintosh computer.

Natural Process Analysis (NPA)

Authors: Shriberg, L., & Kwiatkowski, J. (1980). *Natural Process Analysis*. New York: John Wiley.

Comments: A well-respected test of error patterns for use with children with severely delayed speech; analysis is based on spontaneous speech samples; no specific stimuli are required; requires approximately 1½ hours to administer.

Phonological Assessment of Child Speech (PACS)

Author: Grunwell, P. (1986). *Phonological Assessment of Child Speech*. Boston, MA: College-Hill Press.

Comments: An impressive comprehensive test for children with multiple error patterns.

Phonological Process Analysis (PPA)

Author: Weiner, F. (1979). *Phonological Process Analysis*. Austin, TX: Pro-Ed.

Comments: Tests 16 error patterns; requires approximately 45 minutes to complete with a cooperative child.

Photo Articulation Test (PAT)

Authors: Pendergast, K., Dickey, S., Selmar, J., & Soder, A. (1969). *Photo Articulation Test*. Danville, IL: Interstate Printers and Publishers.

Comments: A long-time stand-by test of individual sounds for ages 3 through 12 years; pocket-size cards are convenient; requires approximately 15 minutes to complete.

Process Analysis: Version 2.0. [Apple II series computers]

Author: Weiner, F. (1986). *Process Analysis: Version 2.*. State College, PA: Parrot Software.

Comments: Computer version of the PPA designed for Apple computers.

Programs to Examine Phonetic and Phonologic Evaluation Records: Version 4.0. [MS-DOS systems].

Author: Shriberg, L. (1986). *Programs to Examine Phonetic and Phonologic Evaluation Records: Version 4.0.* Hillsdale, NJ: Lawrence Erlbaum.

Comments: Computer version of the highly regarded NPA.

Spanish Articulation Measures (SAM)

Author: Mattes, L. (1993). *Spanish Articulation Measures.* Oceanside, CA: Academic Communication Associates.

Comments: Assesses Spanish-speaking children's acquisition of individual sounds and elimination of error patterns.

The Templin-Darley Tests of Articulation (Templin-Darley)

Authors: Templin, M., & Darley, F. (1969). *The Templin-Darley Tests of Articulation.* Iowa City: University of Iowa Bureau of Educational Research and Service.

Comments: A classic test of individual sounds for late preschoolers and school-age children.

Test of Minimal Articulation Competence (T-MAC)

Author: Secord, W. (1981). *Test of Minimal Articulation Competence.* San Antonio, TX: The Psychological Corporation.

Comments: A traditional test of individual sounds; requires approximately 10–20 minutes to complete.

Test of Phonological Awareness (TOPA)

Authors: Torgesen, J., & Bryant, B. (1994). *Test of Phonological Awareness.* Austin, TX: Pro-Ed.

Comments: A new test of a child's awareness of individual sounds in words.

Weiss Comprehensive Articulation Test (WCAT)

Author: Weiss, C. (1980). *Weiss Comprehensive Articulation Test.* Chicago, IL: Riverside.

Comments: A well-respected test for preschoolers to adults.

VII. RELATED ASSESSMENTS

Other aspects of a complete speech-language evaluation can have an important influence on the articulation and phonological assessment.

A. Language Assessment

The language assessment (especially information on language reception abilities) helps establish the client's upper potential for articulation and phonological development. In most cases, a child 10 years of age with mental retardation, whose major language reception abilities approximated a child 3 years of age, for example, would be expected to have (at best) the articulation and phonological abilities of a child 3 years of age. (See Chapter 4 for further discussion of developmental age.)

B. Hearing Screening

The hearing screening establishes whether the client has a hearing impairment that might affect his or her articulation and phonological development.

C. Case History

Several questions asked during the case history can help to determine if the client is either at-risk for an articulation and phonological in the future or presently has an articulation and phonological disorder that is adversely affecting his or her life.

   1. **At-risk Conditions.** At-risk conditions include genetic, medical, and environmental factors. Positive answers to any of the

following questions should alert the clinician that the client may be at-risk for problems in articulation and phonological development:

Does anyone in the client's immediate family have a speech problem?

Does the client have a hearing impairment?

Does the client have any neurological or cognitive handicaps?

Does the client have any medical difficulties or genetic factors that might interfere with present or future articulation and phonological development?

Was the client born more than 4 weeks prematurely?

Does the client have any structural or functional abnormalities of the face or oral motor system?

Is the client a long-term hospital patient?

Has the client experienced neglect?

2. **Effect on Life Situation.** The following questions may serve to determine if speech is adversely affecting the client's life situation.

Ask caregivers of infants and toddlers, "Do you feel that your child has speech problems (problems in vocalizing for infants) that interfere with your interactions?"

Ask caregivers of preschoolers, "Does your child get frustrated when he or she can't be understood?" or "What does your child do when he or she can't be understood?"

Ask late preschoolers and school-age children, "Do people sometimes have trouble understanding you when you talk?" or "If you had three wishes, what would you wish for?" (If the child wishes for better speech or wishes to be understood better, the clinician should consider that a sign for concern.) Alternately, ask the client's caregiver, "Do other children tease your child about his/her speech?"

Ask adults, "Does your speech interfere with your job?" or "How do you feel about your speech?" or "How does your speech affect your life?"

D. Oral Cavity Assessment

The oral cavity assessment helps to determine if the client has gross oral cavity abnormalities that might interfere with speech production (Mason & Wickwire, 1978). The oral cavity assessment requires gloves, a mirror, a penlight, and a tongue depressor. The evaluator should wear gloves, and universal health precautions should be followed. The oral cavity assessment proceeds in the steps below. A sample form for the oral cavity assessment is provided in Appendix 2F.

The Oral Cavity

The speech mechanism is so flexible that persons speak well with high palates, small teeth, a small or large tongue, and many other mild to moderate structural and movement problems. Only the grossest abnormalities are capable of nullifying the human capacity to develop compensatory strategies to minimize physical limitations. If the oral cavity assessment reveals gross abnormalities of structure or movement, the client should be referred to an otolaryngologist, orthodontist, or neurologist.

---

1. **Face.** Sit at eye level across from the client and observe his or her face. Muscle weakness or spasticity might suggest cerebral palsy. Muscle weakness or drooping of one half of the face might suggest paralysis.

2. **Breathing.** Observe the client breathing. Mouth breathing might indicate blockage of the nasal airway. If a problem is suspected, ask the client to close his or her mouth and breathe onto a mirror placed under the nose. An unfogged mirror or inability to breathe through the nose would be additional evidence that the nasal airway is not open.

3. **Lips.** Observe the client's lips for drooling, which might indicate the presence of dysarthria or another oral motor deficiency. Ask the client to perform the following activities to test for movement disorders:

   a. **Spreading.** Ask the client to say [i] (to test lip spreading).

Which Consonant Remains?

When a consonant cluster is reduced, which consonant remains? Typically, but not always, the consonant that remains is the one acquired earlier, according to age norms (see Chapter 3). For example, [st] is likely to be reduced to [t] and [br] is likely to be reduced to [b]. The same principle applies to clusters with three consonants. For example, [spr] is likely to be reduced to either [p] or [sp], whereas the [r], being acquired latest in development of the three sounds, is the consonant most likely to be deleted.

---

    b. **Rounding.** Ask the client to say [u] (to test lip rounding).

    c. **Rapid Movements.** Ask the client to say [pʌpʌpʌ] (to test rapid movements of the lips).

4. **Jaw.** Turn the client's head to each side, and look for gross retrusions or protrusions of the maxilla or mandible.

5. **Teeth.** Ask the client to open his or her mouth so you can examine the teeth.

    a. **Missing Teeth.** Look for missing teeth. Missing front teeth have the most direct effect on speech, especially on [s] and [z].

    b. **Bite.** To observe the client's bite, instruct the client to bite down lightly on the back teeth and to open the lips. In a normal overbite the upper front teeth are about 1/4 inch in front of the lower teeth and cover about one third of the top of the lower teeth.

    c. **Overbite.** Note if the client has an excessive overbite or an open bite (i.e., the upper teeth do not cover part of the lower teeth at any point along the dental arch).

6. Observe the client's tongue.

    a. **Size.** Determine that the tongue is not grossly large or small. A tongue that appears shriveled either on one or both sides might indicate paralysis.

b. **Reach.** Ask the client to touch the alveolar ridge with his or her tongue tip. A client whose tongue tip cannot reach the alveolar ridge may have a short lingual frenum (i.e., the attachment under the tongue).

c. **Laterality.** Instruct the client to move his or her tongue laterally to test its mobility.

7. **Hard Palate.** Instruct the client to extend his or her head back.

a. **Clefts.** Observe the client's hard palate for signs of repaired or unrepaired clefts, fistulas, and fissures.

b. **Coloration.** Observe the midline of the client's hard palate, using a penlight if needed. Normal coloration of the midline is pink and white. A blue tint in the midline could indicate a submucous cleft. A blue tint lateral to the midline is not a cause of alarm. If a blue line is found at the midline, gently rub the posterior portion of the hard palate, feeling for a cleft.

8. **Soft palate.** Instruct the client to open his or her mouth three quarters of maximum to get the best velar elevation.

a. **Clefts.** Observe the soft palate for signs of repaired and unrepaired clefts, fissures, and fistulas.

b. **Coloration.** Look for a normal pink and white coloration at the midline. As with the hard palate, a blue tint at midline may indicate a submucous cleft. A blue tint lateral to the midline is not a cause for concern.

c. **Nasality.** Ask the client to produce a sustained "ah." A nasal sounding "ah" may indicate difficulty closing the nasal tract. Determine whether the client can elevate his or her velum to the plane of the hard palate.

9. **Uvula.** Ask the client to say a sustained "ah" and observe his or her uvula. A bifid uvula (it looks like two uvula) might indicate the presence of other anatomical problems.

10. **Fauces.** Ask the client to say a sustained "ah" and look for signs of redness, inflammation, or movement of the faucial pillars that might indicate infection.

11. **Pharynx.** Ask the client to say a sustained "ah" and look at the back of his or her throat. Presence of a Passavant's pad might indicate a possible velopharyngeal valving problem.

APPENDIX 2A
Sample Screening Items

A. Introduction

To screen for articulation and phonological disorders, (1) obtain a short spontaneous speech sample to help develop an initial impression of the client's level of intelligibility or severity of involvement and (2) elicit the underlined sounds shown on the following pages. The typical ages at which the underlined sounds are acquired are listed in parentheses (Smit, Hand, Frelinger, Bernthal, & Byrd, 1990). To illustrate the information gathering procedure, a spontaneous speech sample might be obtained by asking, "What did you have for breakfast?" To elicit the underlined sounds, a client aged 4;10, for example, would be asked to say the words in Category C, the closest category below the client's chronological age. Clients older than 5 years of age are compared to the age norms in Category D. A client is placed within a category based on developmental age instead of chronological age if a intellectual limitations or a cognitive impairment exists. Clients with no risk factors (see Section VII) who miss more than one underlined sound should be referred for a complete articulation and phonological assessment. Clients with risk factors (see Section VII) should be referred for a complete evaluation if they miss one underlined sound.

B. Elicitation Procedures

Elicit either isolated words or sentences using the phrase, "Repeat after me: _____ . Now you say it." If the client answers too quickly, say "First wait for me to finish," followed by repetition of the word or sentence.

Example

Begin the screening with an example of the procedure.

Isolated word: "Repeat after me: dog. Now you say it."

Sentence: "Repeat after me: The man walked home. Now you say it." If the client answers too quickly, say "First wait for me to finish," followed by repetition of the sample.

Sample Screening Items

A. For Clients 3;6–3;11

t̲win	_____	(3;0)
q̲uick	_____	(3;0)
s̲on	_____	(3;6)
z̲oo	_____	(3;6)
s̲kip	_____	(3;6)
p̲lay	_____	(3;6)

Or: "My t̲win is q̲uick." (3;0)
    "My s̲on p̲lays at the z̲oo." (3;6)

B. For Clients 4;0–4;5

s̲on	_____	(3;6)
z̲oo	_____	(3;6)
s̲kip	_____	(3;6)
p̲lay	_____	(3;6)
p̲lea̲se	_____	(4;0)
p̲ride	_____	(4;0)
d̲ry	_____	(4;0)
c̲rowd	_____	(4;0)

Or: "My s̲on p̲lays at the z̲oo." (3;6)
    "Plea̲se don't make the baby c̲ry." (4;0)

C. For Clients 4;6–4;11

p̲lease	_____	(4;0)
p̲ride	_____	(4;0)

dry   _____   (4;0)

crowd   _____   (4;0)

thumb   _____   (4;6)

grape   _____   (4;6)

slip   _____   (4;6)

Or: "Please don't make the baby cry." (4;0)
     "The boy slipped on a grape." (4;6)

D. For Clients 5 Years or Older

thumb   _____   (4;6)

grape   _____   (4;6)

slip   _____   (4;6)

tree   _____   (5;0)

spring   _____   (5;0)

string   _____   (5;0)

splash   _____   (5;0)

Or: "The boy slipped on a grape. (4;6)
     "The water splashed on a tree." (5;0)

APPENDIX 2B
Word Probes for Consonants,
Consonant Clusters, and [ɚ]

A. Introduction

The following sound probes are used either during the initial elicitation or follow-up hypothesis testing to help determine whether a client in Stage 3 or Stage 4 is able to produce a sound correctly. The sound probes may also be used to test for stimulability, key phonetic environments, key words (see Section V in Chapter 3) and for pre- and post-testing (see Chapter 4). To illustrate, stimulability of [s] might be tested by asking the client to repeat the sound lists for [s]. Similarly, a pretest for [k] might be obtained by having the client say the word list for [k] at the onset of treatment, and a post-test might be obtained by having the client say the same sound list after the client is thought to have learned how to produce [k]. The sound probes that follow test consonants, consonant clusters, and [ɚ] in the most commonly tested phonetic environments: word initially, between syllables (between vowels when possible), and word finally. Most often, five words for each sound are presented, although fewer words are used for several sounds for which it was harder to find words. The clinician should create additional probes to test more words and different phonetic environments, as the need arises.

B. Procedures

Elicit the words through naming, sentence completion, delayed imitation, or imitation. Transcribe the entire word if the client is in Stage 3; transcribe isolated sounds if the client is in Stage 4. To determine the sounds for which a client is stimulable, have the client imitate a sound and place a check mark next to sounds the client imitates correctly.

Word Probes for Consonants, Consonant Clusters, and [ɚ]

Oral Stops

[p]

# ___		s ___ s		___ #	
pan	___	puppy	___	mop	___
pot	___	papa	___	map	___
pony	___	diaper	___	hop	___
pie	___	muppet	___	pop	___
pin	___	sleepy	___	ape	___

[b]

# ___		s ___ s		___ #	
bee	___	baby	___	crab	___
bat	___	Abby	___	bib	___
book	___	hobo	___	tub	___
boot	___	hobby	___	fib	___
bike	___	tuba	___	web	___

[t]

# ___		s ___ s		___ #	
tea	___	Patty	___	ate	___
tail	___	water	___	bat	___
toe	___	waiter	___	pot	___
tie	___	twenty	___	foot	___
tag	___	Rita	___	boat	___

[d]

# ___		s ___ s		___ #	
dive	___	daddy	___	kid	___
dog	___	soda	___	mud	___
doll	___	caddy	___	bed	___
dot	___	Sunday	___	sad	___
dam	___	birdie	___	head	___

(continued)

Oral Stops (continued)

[k]

# __		S __ S		__ #	
key	___	bucket	___	bike	___
cat	___	lucky	___	sick	___
kite	___	broken	___	duck	___
coat	___	sneaky	___	book	___
candy	___	icky	___	peek	___

[g]

# __		S __ S		__ #	
gum	___	buggy	___	bag	___
good	___	tiger	___	leg	___
guy	___	wiggle	___	frog	___
goat	___	piggy	___	big	___
go	___	groggy	___	dog	___

Fricatives and Affricates

Fricatives

[f]

# __		S __ S		__ #	
fun	___	sniffle	___	safe	___
feet	___	taffy	___	hoof	___
fire	___	sofa	___	knife	___
fog	___	gopher	___	cough	___
face	___	offer	___	off	___

[v]

# __		S __ S		__ #	
vine	___	movie	___	dove	___
van	___	navy	___	live	___
vote	___	lava	___	wave	___
very	___	diver	___	brave	___
valley	___	never	___	move	___

[θ]

#	S_S	_#
think	nothing	teeth
thief	panther	with
thumb	something	north
thick	author	mouth
thanks	Kathy	broth

[s]

#	S_S	_#
sun	icy	bus
soap	messy	kiss
sit	castle	face
say	bossy	hiss
see	messy	horse

[ʃ]

#	S_S	_#
shoe	wishing	dish
sheep	ocean	crash
shiny	washer	wash
shut	fishy	wish
shell	dishes	splash

[ð]

#	S_S
that	weather
this	feather
them	brother
then	either
these	neither

[z]

#	S_S	_#
zoo	daisy	keys
zero	busy	please
zoom	freezer	buzz
zip	lizard	news
zebra	music	eyes

[ʒ]

S_S	_#
Asia	garage
vision	beige
leisure	treasure
measure	
seizure	

(continued)

Fricatives and Affricates (continued)

Affricates

[tʃ]

#___		S___S		___#	
chair	___	itchy	___	watch	___
chew	___	teacher	___	peach	___
chain	___	matches	___	witch	___
cheese	___	nature	___	catch	___
chase	___	pitching	___	ouch	___
cheep	___	watching	___	speech	___

[dʒ]

#___		S___S		___#	
jump	___	magic	___	judge	___
jet	___	cages	___	huge	___
juice	___	edges	___	page	___
joy	___	ranger	___	cage	___
jar	___	danger	___	badge	___
joke	___	ages	___	stage	___

Liquids, Glides, and [ɝ]

[r]

#___		S___S		___#	
rain	___	story	___	car	___
row	___	marry	___	air	___
root	___	hero	___	chair	___
run	___	very	___	bear	___
ring	___	arrow	___	boar	___

Liquids

[l]

#___		S___S		___#	
light	___	pillow	___	ball	___
laugh	___	sailor	___	fall	___
left	___	valley	___	eel	___
lie	___	alley	___	doll	___
low	___	balloon	___	yell	___

[w]

#___

wind	___
we	___
web	___
win	___
wet	___

s___s

flower	___
rowing	___
tower	___
growing	___
shower	___

[j]

#___

yes	___
yard	___
you	___
used	___
yell	___

s___s

crayon	___
million	___
onion	___
billion	___
Mayo	___

[h]

#___

home	___
he	___
hat	___
hi	___
help	___

[ɚ]

C___C

worm	___
girl	___
bird	___
shirt	___
burn	___

C___#

fur	___
her	___
tower	___
over	___
pepper	___

(continued)

Nasal Stops

[m]

#___	S___S	___#
moon	gummy	dam
me	comet	boom
mud	mummy	aim
mop	mama	swim
meat	hammer	game

[n]

#___	S___S	___#
nice	running	spoon
no	honey	pan
knife	winner	train
nut	rainy	can
new	tiny	fun

[ŋ]

S___S	___#
hanger	hang
singing	sing
finger	bang
winging	wing
clanging	king

Consonant Clusters

[l] Clusters

[pl]

# __	S __ S
play	airplane
plate	apply
please	applaud
place	
plane	

[kl]

# __	S __ S
clock	duckling
cloud	ticklish
clue	weekly
class	
clap	

[bl]

# __	S __ S
bloom	ably
blind	cobbler
blood	wobbling
blow	
blank	

[gl]

# __	S __ S
glue	giggling
glow	ugly
gloomy	burgler
glass	
glad	

[fl]

# __	S __ S
flag	cornflake
fly	snowflake
floor	stiffly
flower	
flip	

[sl]

# __	S __ S
slam	wrestler
sleep	asleep
slow	nicely
slip	
sleigh	

(continued)

85

Consonant Clusters (continued)

[r] Clusters

[pr]

#		s___s	
pretty	___	suprise	___
print	___	supreme	___
prune	___	apron	___
pray	___		
praise	___		

[br]

#		s___s	
brain	___	umbrella	___
branch	___	fabric	___
break	___	library	___
broom	___		
bright	___		

[tr]

#		s___s	
trout	___	country	___
truck	___	subtract	___
tree	___	pantry	___
tray	___		
treat	___		

[dr]

#		s___s	
dry	___	address	___
drink	___	laundry	___
drop	___	raindrop	___
drum	___		
dress	___		

[kr]

#		s___s	
crib	___	secret	___
crow	___	across	___
cry	___	recruit	___
crowd	___		
cream	___		

[gr]

#		s___s	
grin	___	regret	___
grill	___	agree	___
grow	___	photograph	___
great	___		
grass	___		

[r] Clusters

[fr]
#___

fruit	___
free	___
fried	___
great	___
freeze	___

s___s

defrost	___
afraid	___
refreshment	___

[θr]
#___

three	___
throw	___
thread	___

[w] Clusters

[tw]
#___

twin	___
twice	___
twig	___
twilight	___
twirl	___

[kw]
#___

quit	___
queen	___
quake	___
quiet	___
quick	___

[sw]
(see [s] clusters)

(continued)

Consonant Clusters *(continued)*

[s] Clusters

[sp]

#___	S___S	___#
spill	whisper	wasp
space	inspect	lisp
spy	gospel	crisp
spark		
spin		

[st]

#___	S___S	___#
stove	mustard	most
stew	rooster	last
star	faster	lost
storm		
stop		

[sk]

#___	S___S	___#
sky	basket	ask
skip	scooter	mask
ski	risky	task
skunk		
skate		

[sw]

#___	S___S
swamp	upswing
swim	high swing
sweet	carpet sweeper
sweater	
swell	

[sm]
 # ___
smell _____
smoke _____
smile _____
small _____
smart _____

s___s
iceman _____
goldsmith _____
basement _____
_____
_____

[sn]
s___s
snow _____
snail _____
snap _____
snake _____
snack _____

s___s
unsnap _____
closeness _____
looseness _____

[sl]
(see [l] clusters)

[spr]
 # ___
spray _____
spread _____
spring _____
sprint _____
sprinkle _____

[str]
 # ___
strap _____
straw _____
stream _____
strange _____
street _____

[skr]
 # ___
scream _____
scratch _____
screen _____
screw _____
scrap _____

[skw]
 # ___
squirrel _____
square _____
squad _____
squeak _____
squirt _____

[spl]
 # ___
splash _____
splendid _____
splatter _____
split _____
splurge _____

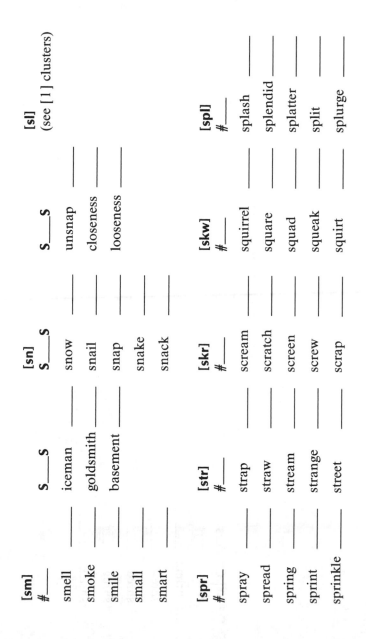

(continued)

Consonant Clusters *(continued)*

[ʃr] Clusters

#_____

shrimp _____

shrew _____

shred _____

shrug _____

shriek _____

APPENDIX 2C
Word Probes for Error Patterns

A. Introduction

The error probes that follow test 23 error patterns that, together, account for most error patterns found in speech of clients in Stages 2 and 3. The most common error patterns are indicated with triple stars (***). The error probes are primarily used during the initial elicitation or during follow-up hypothesis testing. Error probes can also be used to test for stimulability, key phonetic environments, key words (see Section V in Chapter 3), and for pre- and post-testing (see Chapter 4). If the clinician wishes, additional error probes can be developed either to test different error patterns or to test an error pattern in more depth. To illustrate the latter situation, the error probes for the Lisping pattern test alveolar fricatives but not postalveolar fricatives which sometimes also are affected. To determine if a particular client's lisping pattern also affects postalveolar fricatives (and other consonants as well, if warranted), the clinician could develop words containing fricatives produced at other places of production. A form to help summarize information from error probes is provided in Appendix 3L.

B. Procedures

The speediest procedure to elicit the words is through delayed imitation or imitation, which allows stimulability to be determined at the same time as the words are elicited (see Chapter 3 for a discussion of stimulability). If the words are elicited through naming or sentence completion, stimulability can be determined afterwards by asking the client to imitate words displaying the error patterns.

The examples on the following pages illustrates how word probes for error patterns might be utilized to assess Fronting. Delayed imitation was used to elicit the words, and, therefore, additional stimulability testing was not undertaken.

Example: Fronting***

Definition: Substitution of an alveolar stop for a velar or postalveolar consonant.

Focus: Listen to the velar and postalveolar consonants. If they are said as alveolar consonants, the client likely has a Fronting pattern.

Word	Transcription	Yes/No	(Stimulable)
key	t k̸i	X	NA*
cheap	tʃip	—	NA
bug	d bʌg̸	X	NA
bush	bʊʃ	—	NA
itch	ɪtʃ	—	NA
pick	pɪk	—	NA
sheep	s ʃ̸ip	X	NA
jump	dʒʌmp	—	NA
go	goʊ	—	NA
edge	ɛdʒ	—	NA
Total		3/10	—

***Triple stars indicate the most common error patterns.

1. **Definition.** The error probe begins with a definition of the error pattern.

2. **Focus.** The focus statement indicates the particular aspects of the client's speech to which the clinicians should attend.

3. **Word.** The words used to elicit the error pattern are listed on the left. The sounds that the error pattern may affect are underlined.

4. **Transcription.** The transcription is listed in the column next to the elicited words. Sounds affected by the error pattern are crossed out, and the client's production is indicated above the crossed out sound.

5. **Yes/No.** A check mark indicates that the pattern was elicited and a dash indicates the pattern was not elicited. The checks are totaled at the bottom, being careful to total only errors that result from the error pattern. Error patterns occurring approximately 40% of the time (2 or more times out of 5 opportunities or 4 out of 10 opportunities) are likely short-term treatment goals (see Chapter 4).

6. **Stimulability.** If the words are not elicited through delayed or immediate imitation, the client's stimulability for the sound is indicated through a check mark in the last column.

Word Probes for Error Patterns

A. Changes in Place of Production

1. Fronting***

Definition: Substitution of an alveolar stop for a postalveolar or velar consonant.

Focus: Listen to the underlined postalveolar and velar consonants. If they are said as alveolar consonants, the client likely has a Fronting pattern.

Word	Transcription	Yes/No	(Stimulable)
key	ki	_____	_____
cheap	tʃip	_____	_____
bug	bʌg	_____	_____
bush	bʊʃ	_____	_____
itch	ɪtʃ	_____	_____
pick	pɪk	_____	_____
sheep	ʃip	_____	_____
jump	dʒʌmp	_____	_____
go	goʊ	_____	_____
edge	ɛdʒ	_____	_____
Total		___/___	_____

2. Lisping***

Definition: Alveolar consonants (especially fricatives) are pronounced either on or between the teeth; may also be produced with air flowing over the sides of the tongue, in which case it is called a lateral lisp.

Focus: Listen to the underlined alveolar fricatives. If they are pronounced either on or between the teeth, the client likely has a Lisping pattern. If the air flows over the sides of the tongue, the client has a Lateral Lisping pattern.

Word	Transcription	Yes/No	(Stimulable)
zoo	zu	_____	_____
bus	bʌs	_____	_____
zero	zirou	_____	_____
ozone	ouzoun	_____	_____
sun	sʌn	_____	_____
sneeze	sniz	_____	_____
asleep	əslip	_____	_____
see	si	_____	_____
maze	meɪz	_____	_____
easy	izi	_____	_____
Total:		__/__	_____

3. Velar Assimilation***

Definition: Consonants assimilate to the place of production of a velar consonant.

Focus: Listen to the unerlined non-velar consonants. If they are said as velar consonants, the client likely has a Velar Assimilation pattern.

Word	Transcription	Yes/No	(Stimulable)
bug	bʌg	_____	_____
cup	kʌp	_____	_____
duck	dʌk	_____	_____
poke	poʊk	_____	_____
goat	goʊt	_____	_____
pig	pɪg	_____	_____
beak	bik	_____	_____
dig	dɪg	_____	_____
kite	kaɪt	_____	_____
tag	tæg	_____	_____
Total		__/__	_____

4. Labial Assimilation***

Definition: Consonants assimilate to the place of production of a labial consonant.

Focus: Listen to the underlined non-labial consonants. If the consonants are said as labial consonants, the client likely has a Labial Assimilation pattern.

Word	Transcription	Yes/No	(Stimulable)
bug	bʌg	_____	_____
cup	kʌp	_____	_____
tape	teɪp	_____	_____
dip	dɪp	_____	_____
deep	dip	_____	_____
bite	baɪt	_____	_____
cape	keɪp	_____	_____
pig	pɪg	_____	_____
beak	bik	_____	_____
cab	kæb	_____	_____
Total:		___/___	_____

5. Backing

Definition: Alveolar (and sometimes postalveolar) consonants are pronounced as velar stops.

Focus: Listen to the underlined alveolar and psotalveolar consonants. If they are said as velar stops, the client likely has a Backing pattern.

Word	Transcription	Yes/No	(Stimulable)
tie	taɪ	_____	_____
bus	bʌs	_____	_____
kid	kɪd	_____	_____
bush	bʊʃ	_____	_____
day	deɪ	_____	_____
see	si	_____	_____
itch	ɪtʃ	_____	_____
eat	it	_____	_____
zoo	zu	_____	_____
jump	dʒʌmp	_____	_____
Total:		___/___	_____

6. Glottal replacement

Definition: Replacement of a consonant with a glottal stop.

Focus: Listen to the underlined consonants. If they are said as glottal stops, the client likely has a Glottal Replacement pattern.

Word	Transcription	Yes/No	(Stimulable)
bug	bʌg	_____	_____
up	ʌp	_____	_____
little	lıfl	_____	_____
key	ki	_____	_____
baby	beɪbi	_____	_____
beetle	bifl	_____	_____
funny	fʌni	_____	_____
jet	dʒɛt	_____	_____
package	pækɪdʒ	_____	_____
egg	eɪg	_____	_____
Total:		__/__	_____

B. Changes in Manner of Production

1. Stopping***

Definition: Substitution of a stop for a fricative or affricate.

Focus: Listen to the underlined fricatives and affricates. If an underlined consonant is said as a stop, the client likely has a Stopping pattern.

Word	Transcription	Yes/No	(Stimulable)
su̲n	sʌn	_____	_____
f̲un	fʌn	_____	_____
bu̲s	bʌs	_____	_____
t̲hin	θɪn	_____	_____
j̲oke	dʒoʊk	_____	_____
z̲oo	zu	_____	_____
div̲e	daɪv	_____	_____
maz̲e	meɪz	_____	_____
c̲himp	tʃɪmp	_____	_____
s̲hip	ʃɪp	_____	_____
Total:		___/___	_____

2. Gliding***

Definition: Substitution of a glide for a liquid.

Focus: Listen to the underlined liquid consonants. If they are said as glides, the client likely has a Gliding pattern.

Word	Transcription	Yes/No	(Stimulable)
rain	reɪn	_____	_____
light	laɪt	_____	_____
run	rʌn	_____	_____
row	roʊ	_____	_____
log	lɔg	_____	_____
leaf	lif	_____	_____
ring	rɪŋ	_____	_____
low	loʊ	_____	_____
ray	reɪ	_____	_____
late	leɪt	_____	_____
Total		___/___	_____

3. Lateralization***

Definition: Sounds typically produced with central air emission (most commonly [s] and [z], but sometimes [ʃ], [ʒ], [tʃ], and [dʒ]) are pronounced with lateral air emission.

Focus: Listen to the underlined consonants. If they are pronounced with lateral air emission, the client likely has a lateralization pattern.

Word	Transcription	Yes/No	(Stimulable)
zoo	zu	_____	_____
buş	bʌs	_____	_____
cheap	tʃip	_____	_____
zero	zirou	_____	_____
sun	sʌn	_____	_____
beach	bitʃ	_____	_____
show	ʃou	_____	_____
sneeze	sniz	_____	
bush	buʃ	_____	_____
joke	dʒouk	_____	_____
Total:		__/__	_____

4. Affrication

Definition: Stops or fricatives (both usually alveolars) are pronounced as affricates.

Focus: Listen to the underlined stops and fricatives. If they are pronounced as affricates, the client likely has an Affrication pattern.

Word	Transcription	Yes/No	(Stimulable)
sun	sʌn	_____	_____
mat	mæt	_____	_____
city	sɪʃi	_____	_____
bus	bʌs	_____	_____
day	deɪ	_____	_____
toe	toʊ	_____	_____
maze	meɪz	_____	_____
mad	mæd	_____	_____
daisy	deɪzi	_____	_____
zoo	zu	_____	_____
Total:		__/__	_____

5. Nasalization

Definition: Non-nasal consonants (usually oral stops) are pronounced as nasal stops.

Focus: Listen to the underlined oral stops. If they are said as nasal stops, the client likely has a Nasalization pattern.

Word	Transcription	Yes/No	(Stimulable)
bug	bʌg	_____	_____
bee	bi	_____	_____
pie	paɪ	_____	_____
go	goʊ	_____	_____
kite	kaɪt	_____	_____
lid	lɪd	_____	_____
sheep	ʃip	_____	_____
day	deɪ	_____	_____
coat	koʊt	_____	_____
peek	pik	_____	_____
Total:		__/__	_____

6. Denasalization

Definition: Nasal consonants are pronounced as oral consonants (usually oral stops).

Focus: Listen to the underlined nasal consonants. If they are said as oral stops, the client likely has a Denasalization pattern.

Word	Transcription	Yes/No	(Stimulable)
mud	mʌd	_____	_____
song	sɔŋ	_____	_____
nap	næp	_____	_____
may	meɪ	_____	_____
name	neɪm	_____	_____
wing	wiŋ	_____	_____
lamb	læm	_____	_____
new	nu	_____	_____
moon	mun	_____	_____
sun	sʌn	_____	_____
Total:		___/___	_____

C. Changes in the Beginning of Syllables or Words

1. Prevocalic Voicing***

Definition: Consonants are voiced when occurring before a vowel.

Focus: Listen to the underlined, word-initial consonants. If they are said with voicing, the client likely has a Prevocalic Voicing pattern.

Word	Transcription	Yes/No	(Stimulable)
pie	paɪ	_____	_____
show	ʃoʊ	_____	_____
toe	toʊ	_____	_____
thin	θɪn	_____	_____
key	ki	_____	_____
top	tɑp	_____	_____
see	ʃi		
fun	fʌn	_____	_____
cold	koʊld	_____	_____
Total:		___/___	_____

2. Initial Consonant Deletion

Definition: The initial consonant in the word is deleted.

Focus: Listen to the underlined, word-initial consonants. If they are deleted, the client likely has an Initial Consonant Devoicing pattern.

Word	Transcription	Yes/No	(Stimulable)
bee	bi	_____	_____
zoo	zu	_____	_____
cow	kaʊ	_____	_____
sun	sʌn	_____	_____
kite	kaɪt	_____	_____
fun	fʌn	_____	_____
pea	pi	_____	_____
go	goʊ	_____	_____
sheep	ʃip	_____	_____
thin	θɪn	_____	_____
Total:		__/__	_____

D. Changes at the End of Syllables or Words

1. Final Consonant Devoicing***

Definition: Obstruents are voiceless at the ends of words.

Focus: Listen to the underlined, word-final consonants. If they are said without voicing, the client likely has a Final Consonant Devoicing pattern.

Word	Transcription	Yes/No	(Stimulable)
bu<u>zz</u>	bʌz	_____	_____
pi<u>g</u>	pɪg	_____	_____
su<u>b</u>	sʌb	_____	_____
mu<u>d</u>	mʌd	_____	_____
ca<u>ve</u>	keɪv	_____	_____
e<u>dge</u>	ɛdʒ	_____	_____
brea<u>the</u>	brið	_____	_____
mu<u>g</u>	mʌg	_____	_____
bi<u>d</u>	bɪd	_____	_____
ro<u>be</u>	roʊb	_____	_____
Total:		___/___	_____

2. Final Consonant Deletion***

Definition: Deletion of a consonant at the end of a syllable or word.

Focus: Listen to the underlined, word-final consonants. If they are deleted, the client likely has a Final Consonant Deletion pattern.

Word	Transcription	Yes/No	(Stimulable)
sto<u>p</u>	stɑp	_____	_____
bu<u>s</u>	bʌs	_____	_____
ca<u>ve</u>	keɪv	_____	_____
bi<u>g</u>	bɪg	_____	_____
bi<u>b</u>	bɪb	_____	_____
ki<u>ng</u>	kiŋ	_____	_____
bu<u>zz</u>	bʌz	_____	_____
smo<u>ke</u>	smoʊk	_____	_____
bu<u>sh</u>	bʊʃ	_____	_____
bea<u>ch</u>	bitʃ	_____	_____
Total:		___/___	_____

E. Changes in Syllables

1. Reduplication***

Definition: Repetition of a syllable.

Focus: Listen to the underlined syllables. If they are repeated, the client likely has a Reduplication pattern.

Word	Transcription	Yes/No	(Stimulable)
<u>wa</u>ter	wɑʃɚ	_____	_____
<u>ca</u>rrot	kɛɪt	_____	_____
<u>ki</u>tty	kɪʃi	_____	_____
<u>ba</u>by	beɪbi	_____	_____
<u>su</u>nny	sʌni	_____	_____
<u>bu</u>nny	bʌni	_____	_____
<u>ye</u>llow	jɛloʊ	_____	_____
<u>bu</u>tter	bʌʃɚ	_____	_____
<u>do</u>ggy	dɔgi	_____	_____
<u>coo</u>kie	kʊki	_____	_____
Total:		___/___	_____

2. Syllable Deletion***

Definition: Deletion of an unstressed syllable.

Focus: Listen to the underlined syllables. If they are deleted, the client likely has a Syllable Deletion pattern.

Word	Transcription	Yes/No	(Stimulable)
banana	bənænə	_____	_____
balloon	bəlun	_____	_____
money	mʌni	_____	_____
afraid	əfreɪd	_____	_____
below	bilou	_____	_____
water	wɑʃɚ	_____	_____
kitty	kɪʃi	_____	_____
spaghetti	spəgɛʃi	_____	_____
bunny	bʌni	_____	_____
yellow	jɛlou	_____	_____
Total:		___/___	_____

F. Changes in Consonant Clusters

1. Cluster Reduction***

Definition: Deletion of a consonant in a consonant cluster.

Focus: Listen to the underlined consonant clusters. If one of the consonants is deleted, the client likely has a Cluster Reduction pattern.

Word	Transcription	Yes/No	(Stimulable)
stop	stɑp	_____	_____
bright	braɪt	_____	_____
slide	slaɪd	_____	_____
fix	fɪks	_____	_____
burnt	bɚnt	_____	_____
queen	kwin	_____	_____
spray	spreɪ	_____	_____
pride	praɪd		
twin	twɪn	_____	_____
mist	mɪst	_____	_____
Total:		__/__	_____

Which Consonant Remains?

When a consonant cluster is reduced, which consonant remains? Typically, but not always, the consonant that remains is the one that is acquired earlier, according to age norms (see Chapter 3). For example, [st] is likely to be reduced to [t] and [br] is likely to be reduced to [b]. The same principle applies to clusters with three consonants. For example, [spr] is likely to be reduced to either [p] or [sp], whereas the [r], being acquired latest in the development of the three sounds, is the consonant most likely to be deleted.

2. Epenthesis (ePENthesis)***

Definition: Insertion of a vowel between consonants in a consonant cluster.

Focus: Listen to the underlined consonant clusters. If a schwa appears between the consonants, the client likely has an Epenthesis pattern.

Word	Transcription	Yes/No	(Stimulable)
smile	sməɪl	_____	_____
please	pliz	_____	_____
fry	fraɪ	_____	_____
drain	dreɪn	_____	_____
pray	preɪ	_____	_____
queen	kwin	_____	_____
stop	stɑp	_____	_____
sleep	slip	_____	_____
train	treɪn	_____	_____
spray	spreɪ	_____	_____
Total:		___/___	_____

G. Sound Reversals

1. Metathesis (meTAthesis)

Definition: The reversal of two sounds in a word, for example, saying "pet" as "tep."

Focus: Listen to the underlined consonants. If the consonants are reversed in word-position, the client likely has a Metathesis error.

Word	Transcription	Yes/No	(Stimulable)
bug	bʌg	_____	_____
open	oʊpɪn	_____	_____
sun	sʌn	_____	_____
kite	kaɪt	_____	_____
goat	goʊt	_____	_____
deep	dip	_____	_____
sheep	ʃip	_____	_____
comb	koʊm	_____	_____
fun	fʌn	_____	_____
big	bɪg	_____	_____
Total:		__/__	_____

Influence of Dialect

Many persons who speak African American dialects pronounce [sk] in "ask" as [ks]. This pattern is the result of dialect, not a metathesis pattern.

H. Changes in Vowels and Syllabic Consonants

1. Vowel Neutralization***

Definition: A vowel is replaced with a neutral vowel (schwa, [ʊ], or [ɪ]).

Focus: Listen to the underlined words. If the vowels are said as a neutral vowel (schwa, [ʊ], or [ɪ]), the client likely has a Vowel Neutralization Pattern.

Word	Transcription	Yes/No	(Stimulable)
bee	bi	_____	_____
cat	kæt	_____	_____
kite	kaɪt	_____	_____
dog	dɔg	_____	_____
sat	sæt	_____	_____
sheep	ʃip	_____	_____
big	bɪg	_____	_____
comb	koʊm	_____	_____
goat	goʊt	_____	_____
grape	greɪp	_____	_____
Total:		___/___	_____

2. Vocalization***

Definition: A syllabic consonant is replaced by a neutral vowel (schwa, [ʊ], or [ɪ]).

Focus: Listen to the underlined syllabic consonants. If they are said as a neutral vowel (schwa, [ʊ], or [ɪ]), the client likely has a Vocalization pattern.

Word	Transcription	Yes/No	(Stimulable)
zipp<u>er</u>	zɪpɚ	_____	_____
sadd<u>en</u>	sædn	_____	_____
teach<u>er</u>	titʃɚ	_____	_____
bott<u>le</u>	baʃl	_____	_____
bigg<u>er</u>	bɪgɚ	_____	_____
sadd<u>le</u>	sædl	_____	_____
bott<u>om</u>	baʃm	_____	_____
catt<u>le</u>	kæʃl	_____	_____
butt<u>on</u>	bʌɪn̊	_____	_____
ratt<u>le</u>	ræʃl	_____	_____
Total:		___/___	_____

APPENDIX 2D
Multiple Error Patterns

A. Introduction

More than one error pattern can affect a sound.Three common error patterns often involved in multiple error patterns are Stopping, Prevocalic Voicing, and Final Consonant Devoicing. The following tables illustrate how these patterns combine with each other and with three other common error patterns — Fronting, Cluster Reduction, and Epenthesis. Sounds typically affected by the patterns appear on the left, and the pronunciations of the sound as it undergoes various patterns are depicted on the right. An example is included in each table to illustrate the effects of multiple patterns on words.

B. Stopping and Prevocalic Voicing

Sounds	Stopping	+ Prevocalic Voicing
feet [fit]	pit	bit
θ	t	d
s	t	d
ʃ	t	d
tʃ	t	d

C. Stopping and Final Consonant Devoicing

Sounds	Stopping	+ Final Consonant Devoicing
eve [iv]	ib	ip
ð	d	p
z	d	p
ʒ	d	p
dʒ	d	p

D. Fronting, Stopping, and Prevocalic Voicing

Sounds	Fronting	+	Stopping	+	Prevocalic Voicing
keep [kip]	tip		—		dip
ʃ	s		t		d
tʃ	s or t		t		d

E. Consonant Cluster Reduction, Stopping, and Prevocalic Voicing

Sample Clusters	Cluster Reduction	+	Stopping	+	Prevocalic Voicing
fleet [flit]	fit		pit		bit
fr	f		p		b
sl	s		t		d

F. Epenthesis, Stopping, and Prevocalic Voicing

Sample Clusters	Epenthesis	+	Stopping	+	Prevocalic Voicing
speak [spik]	səpik		təpik		dəbik
fr	fər		pər		bər
sm	səm		təm		dəm
sl	səl		təl		dəl

APPENDIX 2E
Sample Transcription Sheet

Word	Transcription	Environments			Other Environments		
		#___	V___V	___#	___	___	___

APPENDIX 2F
Sample Oral Cavity Assessment Form

A. Instructions

The oral cavity assessment requires gloves, a mirror, a penlight, and a tongue depressor. The evaluator should be gloved, and universal health precautions should be followed. Score each item as "pass" (P) if no abnormal findings are shown, and as "no pass" (NP) if an abnormal finding is discovered. Make comments in the space provided after each item. The following is an example of how an abnormal finding might be indicated.

Example:

P ☐ NP ☒ **1. Face.** Sit at eye level across from the client and observe the face. Muscle weakness or spasticity might suggest cerebral palsy. Muscle weakness or drooping of one-half the face might suggest paralysis.

Comments: drooping left side of face

Sample Oral Cavity Assessment Form

P □ NP □   1. **Face.** Sit at eye level across from the client and observe the face. Muscle weakness or spasticity might suggest cerebral palsy. Muscle weakness or drooping of one-half the face might suggest paralysis.

Comments: _____

P □ NP □   2. **Breathing.** Observe the client breathing. Mouth breathing might indicate blockage of the nasal airway. If a problem is suspected, ask the client to close his or her mouth and breathe onto a mirror placed under the nose. An unfogged mirror or inability to breathe through the nose would be additional evidence that the nasal airway is not open.

Comments: _____

P □ NP □   3. **Lips.** Observe the client's lips for drooling, which might indicate the presence of dysarthria or another oral motor deficiency. Ask the client to perform the following activities to test for movement disorders:

Comments: _____

P □ NP □   a. **Spreading.** Ask the client to say [i] (to test lip spreading).

Comments: _____

P □ NP □   b. **Rounding.** Ask the client to say [u] (to test lip rounding).

Comments: _____

P □ NP □   c. **Rapid Movements.** Ask the client to say [pʌpʌpʌ] (to test rapid movements of the lips).

Comments: _____

P □ NP □   4. **Jaw.** Turn the client's head to each side, observing for gross retrusions or protrusions of the maxilla or mandible.

Comments: _____

P □ NP □   5. **Teeth.** Ask the client to open the mouth so you can examine the teeth.

P ☐ NP ☐   **a. Missing Teeth.** Look for missing teeth. Missing the front teeth have the most direct effect on speech through [s] and [z].

Comments: _____

P ☐ NP ☐   **b. Bite.** To observe the client's bite, instruct the client to bite down lightly on the back teeth and to open the lips. In a normal overbite, the upper front teeth are about 1/4 inch in front of the lower teeth and cover about one third of the top of the lower teeth.

Comments: _____

P ☐ NP ☐   **c. Overbite.** Note whether the client has an excessive overbite or an open bite (i.e., the upper teeth do not cover part of the lower teeth at any point along the dental arch).

Comments: _____

6. Tongue. Observe the client's tongue.

P ☐ NP ☐   **a. Size.** Determine that the tongue is not grossly large or small. A tongue that appears shriveled either on one or both sides might indicate paralysis.

Comments: _____

P ☐ NP ☐   **b. Reach.** Ask the client to touch the alveolar ridge with the tongue tip. A client whose tongue tip cannot reach the alveolar ridge may have a short lingual frenum (i.e., the attachment under the tongue).

Comments: _____

P ☐ NP ☐   **c. Laterality.** Instruct the client to move the tongue laterally to test mobility.

Comments: _____

7. Hard Palate Instruct the client to extend the head back.

P ☐ NP ☐   **a. Clefts.** Observe the hard palate for signs of repaired or unrepaired clefts, fistulas, and fissures.

Comments: _____

P □ NP □   **b. Coloration.** Observe the midline, using a penlight if needed. Normal coloration of the midline is pink and white. A blue tint in the midline could indicate a sub-mucous cleft. A blue tint lateral to the midline is not a cause for alarm. If a blue line is found at the midline, gently rub the posterior portion of the hard palate, feeling for a cleft.

Comments: _____

8. Soft palate. Instruct the client to open his or her mouth three quarters of maximum to get the best velar elevation.

P □ NP □   **a. Clefts.** Observe the soft palate for signs of repaired and unrepaired clefts, fissures, and fistulas.

Comments: _____

P □ NP □   **b. Coloration.** Look for a normal pink and white coloration at the midline. As with the hard palate, a blue tint at midline may indicate a submucous cleft. A blue tint lateral to the midline is not a cause for concern.

Comments: _____

P □ NP □   **c. Nasality.** Ask the client to say a sustained "ah." A nasal sounding "ah" may indicate difficulty closing the nasal tract. Observe to see whether the velum can be elevated to the plane of the hard palate.

Comments: _____

P □ NP □ 9. Uvula. Ask the client to say a sustained "ah" and observe his or her uvula. A bifid uvula (it looks like two uvula) might indicate the presence of other anatomical problems.

Comments: _____

P □ NP □ 10. Fauces. Ask the client to say a sustained "ah" and look for signs of redness and inflammation or movement of the faucial pillars that might indicate infection.

Comments: _____

P ☐ **NP** ☐ **11. Pharynx.** Ask the client to say a sustained "ah" and look at the back of the throat. Presence of a Passavant's Pad might indicate a possible velopharyngeal valving problem.

Comments: _____

CHAPTER

3

Analysis

The following topics are discussed in this chapter:

I. OVERVIEW

Almost all published assessment instruments provide guidelines to help evaluate information obtained during screenings and assessments. Most clinicians, however, prefer to perform their own analyses in addition to those prescribed by standardized tests. The sections in this chapter describe nonstandardized measures of severity, intelligibility, prespeech vocalizations, phonetic inventories, error patterns, individual consonants and consonant clusters, stimulability, phonetic placement and shaping, adjusted and developmental age, dialect, and acquisition strategies. Each section describes specific measures and concludes with brief summary comments. The clinical uses of these types of analysis are summarized in Table 3–1.

Table 3-1. Clinical purposes of five forms of analysis.

Type of Analysis	Clinical Purposes
Severity	A primary means used to establish the need for clinical services
Intelligibility	A possible means to establish the need for clinical services, also a possible means to help select treatment targets
Age norms	A primary means to help select treatment targets, also used to establish the need for clinical services
Better abilities	A primary means to help select treatment targets
Related analyses	A primary means to identify client characteristics important to the articulation and phonological analysis (adjusted age, developmental age, dialect, acquisition strategies)

II. SEVERITY

Severity is a measure of the degree of a client's articulation and phonological disorder. Severity of involvement is a primary measure used to justify providing or refusing clinical treatment. The most frequently used measurement tools assess severity through either clinical judgment scales or percentages.

A. Clinical Judgment Scales of Severity

1. **Appropriate Clients.** Clinical judgment scales are used with clients in all stages to establish the need for treatment, but are most applicable with clients in Stages 3 and 4 for whom clinicians require a quick means to assess large numbers of potential clients.

2. **Description.** The measures used most frequently to assess severity of involvement are clinical judgment scales, which assess severity through the use of judges familiar with the client's speech. The judges typically are one or more speech-language clinicians who are asked to rank the client's articulation and phonological development compared to persons of similar age or level of cognitive development. Sample clin-

ical forms to test for severity using 3- and 4-point scales of clinical judgments are provided in Appendixes 3A and 3B, respectively.

B. Percentage of Consonants Correct (PCC)

1. **Appropriate Clients.** The PCC is used to establish the need for treatment with clients whose speech contains multiple substitutions and deletions. Typically, these clients are in Stage 3.

2. **Description.** As its name suggests, the PCC measures severity as a function of the percentage of consonants the client produces correctly out of the total number of consonants the client attempts (Shriberg & Kwiatkowski, 1982). A sample clinical form and scoring instructions to test for severity using the PCC is provided in Appendix 3C.

C. Articulation Competence Index (ACI)

1. **Appropriate Clients.** The ACI is intended to establish the need for treatment in clients whose speech contains many distortions. Clients include selected children in Stages 3 and 4.

2. **Description.** The ACI is a new measure that was developed to assess the percentage of consonant distortions out of the total number of speech sounds that the client attempts (Shriberg, 1993). Results of a normative study comparing children aged 3;0–5;11 who were without articulation and phonological disorders (N = 199) to children with such disorders (N = 117) indicated that the mean ACI scores of the nondelayed group were under 50%, and the mean scores of the delayed group were near 70% or higher (Shriberg, 1993). A sample clinical form and detailed scoring instructions to test for severity using the ACI are provided in Appendix 3D.

Will My Child Speak?

Some children with developmental disabilities may not learn to speak for many years. A question that often haunts parents of children with this most severe form of articulation and phonological impairment is, will my child ever speak? The general rule of thumb is that if a child is going to speak, he or she will do so by 5 years of age. Every experienced speech-language clinician, however, can point to exceptions to this general rule, remembering children who achieved their first words at somewhat later ages. Further, speech is not all or none. Many more children with disabilities are able to use speech in conjunction with sign language and augmentative communication than do not speak at all (Bleile, 1991a).

D. Percentage of Development

1. **Appropriate Clients.** Percentage of development is used to establish the need for treatment in clients of all levels of articulation and phonological development, but is most useful with clients in Stages 1 through 3.

2. **Description.** Percentage of development is the difference between a client's chronological age and the age equivalent corresponding to his or her level of articulation and phonological development. A child 3 years of age, for example, whose articulation and phonological development approximated that of a child 2 years of age would have a delay of 33%. States differ in the specific cutoff criteria they use to establish the need for articulation and phonological treatment. The State of New Jersey, for example, uses a delay of 33% in one area of development to establish the need for developmental services (Kitley & Buzby-Hadden, 1993). A sample clinical form to test for severity using percentage of development is provided in Appendix 3E.

E. Summary Comments

Severity of involvement is often used to establish the need for articulation and phonological treatment. Unfortunately, severity is determined differently by counties, school districts, and sometimes even by clinicians in the same clinical setting, leading to situations in which a client might be deemed eligible for articulation and phonological services in one community but not in another.

Severity of articulation and phonological involvement is measured by various means, each with its own strengths and limitations. Clinical judgment scales, the most widely used severity assessment instruments, are simple and quick to use, but are highly subjective. The best researched procedure is the PCC, which is intended primarily for use with clients with multiple substitutions and deletions. The value of the PCC is limited somewhat by its dependence on spontaneous speech samples, which makes its use problematic in clinical settings that cannot afford the time needed for data collection and analysis.

The ACI is a new measure of severity intended for use with clients whose speech contains many distortions. A limitation of the ACI is that, as its author notes, reliable databases do not exist to identify various types of distortions (Shriberg, 1993). As with the PCC, the ACI requires a spontaneous speech sample, which limits its potential usefulness in clinical settings that cannot afford the time needed to perform data collection and analysis.

Percentage of development offers a relatively quick means to calculate severity using information that is obtained as part of the evaluation. The developmental theory on which the calculation is based, however, seems somewhat odd, because it is probably more accurate to say that a client's speech is similar to a younger child's speech in some respects rather than saying that the client's speech is a certain percentage younger than a child's chronological age. Percentage of development also appears to ignore individual differences in children's rate of articulation and phonological development.

III. INTELLIGIBILITY

Intelligibility is the factor most frequently cited by both speech-language clinicians and lay persons in deciding the severity of a client's articulation and phonological disorder (Gordon-Brannan, 1994; Shriberg & Kwiatkowski, 1983). Three means used to assess intelligibility are clinical judgment scales of intelligibility, frequency of occurrence, and effects of error patterns on intelligibility.

A Clinical Rule of Thumb

By 3 years of age a child's spontaneous speech should be more than 50% intelligible to unfamiliar adults. By 4 years of age a child's spontaneous speech should be intelligible to unfamiliar adults, even though some articulation and phonological differences between the child's speech and that of the adult community are likely to be present.

A. Clinical Judgment Scales of Intelligibility

1. **Appropriate Clients.** Judgment scales of intelligibility are used with clients in Stages 2 through 4. Like severity scales, intelligibility scales are most useful within clinical settings in which clinicians need to perform large numbers of assessments to identify clients in need of treatment.

2. **Description.** Clinical judgment scales of intelligibility are similar in purpose and method to the clinical judgment scales of severity (see Section II). As with severity judgment scales, a judge or judges (typically, speech-language clinicians) familiar with the client are asked to rank the client's speech compared to persons of similar chronological or developmental age (see Section VI for a discussion of developmental age). Two sample clinical forms for use in testing intelligibility using clinical judgments are provided in Appendixes 3F and 3G.

B. Frequency of Occurrence

1. **Appropriate Clients.** A frequency of occurrence analysis is used with clients in Stages 2 through 4 to help select treatment targets (see Chapter 4).

2. **Description.** Frequency of occurrence refers to the relative frequency of sounds in the language of the client's community. Frequency of occurrence is related to intelligibility based on the hypothesis that, all other matters being equal,

the higher a sound's relative frequency of occurrence the greater the sound's impact on intelligibility. A sample clinical form used to test a client's intelligibility using relative frequency of American English consonants is provided in Appendix 3H.

C. Error Patterns

1. **Appropriate Clients.** Assessment of the effects of error patterns on intelligibility is typically undertaken with clients in Stage 3 to help select short-term goals (see Chapter 4).

2. **Description.** Although clinicians have speculated about the effects of error patterns on intelligibility (Hodson, 1986), the relationship between error patterns and intelligibility has only recently begun to be studied (Leinonen-Davies, 1988; Yavas & Lamprecht, 1988;). A sample error pattern analysis used to assess a client's intelligibility is provided in Appendix 3I. Additionally, research suggests that speakers are more likely to be judged unintelligible as the number of patterns increase, deletion and assimilation patterns increase, unusual patterns occur, patterns co-occur, and variability of patterns increases (Yavas & Lamprecht, 1988).

D. Summary Comments

Intelligibility, although a critical concept in the study of articulation and phonological disorders, is notoriously difficult to measure in clinical settings (Kent et al., 1994). This is because intelligibility does not directly reflect the number of sounds produced correctly. In fact, the correlation between number of consonants produced correctly and perceived intelligibility is relatively low ($r = .42$) (Shriberg & Kwiatkowski, 1982a, 1982b). Factors that affect intelligibility include number of errors, types of errors, consistency of errors, speaking rate, and frequency of the error sound in the language. Intelligibility is also affected by variables that are difficult to control, for example, the listener's familiarity with the speaker and the nature of the social environment in which the speech occurs.

Of the three measures discussed in this section, frequency of occurrence has been studied the most. As with clinical judgment scales of severity, clinical judgment scales of intelligibility are simple and quick to use, but they are highly subjective. The relationship between error patterns and intelligibility has only recently been investigated, and the number of subjects studied to date remains relatively small (Leinonen-Davies, 1988; Yavas & Lamprecht, 1988).

IV. AGE NORMS

Age norms show the average ages at which children without developmental delays acquire articulation and phonological behaviors. Age norms are used to select treatment targets and to establish the age corresponding to the client's articulation and phonological development. A child 4 years of age, for example, whose major articulation and phonological abilities correspond to those of a child 2 years of age, would likely be assessed as having approximately the articulation and phonological skills of a child 2 years of age. In certain treatment approaches, articulation and phonological behaviors that a client is most delayed in acquiring would likely be selected as early treatment targets (see Chapter 4). The areas of development for which age norms are most frequently obtained in clinical settings are prespeech vocalizations, phonetic inventories, error patterns, and consonants and consonant clusters.

A. Prespeech Vocalizations

1. **Appropriate Clients.** Analysis of prespeech vocalizations is undertaken with clients in Stage 1 to help select short-term goals and treatment targets (see Chapter 4) and to establish the age that best approximates the level of the client's articulation and phonological development.

Realistic Criteria

Is a vocalization established if it occurs once? Or does it need to occur three times? Or five times? Or even seven times? Obviously, a criterion of three is likely to identify more vocalizations as established than a criterion of seven. Similarly, in how many words does a sound need

continued

> to occur before we say it is established in a client's pho-
> netic inventory? Once? More than once? Time permit-
> ting, I employ three occurrences as my establishment
> criterion, because I have observed that most clients who
> produce a vocalization or sound three times can pro-
> duce it more frequently in more lengthy evaluations.
> Realistically, however, time does not always permit
> three productions to be obtained. If I use fewer than
> three occurrences to establish a vocalization or sound, I
> indicate this in my clinical report, using a phrase such
> as, "The sound was considered established based on
> two occurrences."

2. **Description.** Prespeech vocalizations are utterances without
apparent meaning that are produced by infants from shortly
after birth to around 11 or 12 months of age (see definition of
independent analysis in Chapter 1, Section III). Many researchers believe that prespeech vocalizations provide "practice" in making the speech mechanism "go where the infant
wants it to go" (Bleile, Stark, & Silverman McGowan, 1993;
Locke, 1983; Locke & Pearson, 1992; Oller, 1980; Stark, 1980;
Vihman, Ferguson, & Elbert, 1986). The client's level of vocal
development is the highest age at which a vocalization occurs three or more times during the evaluation session. A
sample clinical form used to determine the age level that best
approximates the client's prespeech vocalizations is provided in Appendix 3J.

B. Phonetic Inventories

1. **Appropriate Clients.** Analysis of phonetic inventories is
undertaken with clients in Stage 2 and less advanced clients
in Stage 3 to help establish treatment targets (see Chapter 4)
and to determine the age that best approximates the level of
the client's articulation and phonological development.

2. **Description.** Phonetic inventories describe the client's ability to produce speech sounds, regardless of whether or not the
sounds are produced correctly relative to the language of the

client's community (see definition of independent analysis in Chapter 1, Section III). A phonetic inventory analysis, for example, might indicate a client's consonant inventory as containing [t], [k], and [s] but would not indicate whether [t] was produced for [t] in "two" or for [z] in "zebra." The greatest clinical value of a phonetic inventory analysis is that it provides information on the number and types of consonants in phonetic inventories of children during the second and third year of life (Dyson, 1988; Stoel-Gammon, 1985).

The phonetic inventories of children's intelligible utterances are relatively well-documented. However, information that includes both intelligible and unintelligible utterances is based on a smaller number of subjects ($N = 7$) (Robb & Bleile, in press). Sample clinical forms used to perform a phonetic inventory analysis of consonants are provided in Appendix 3K. The developmental level of the client's phonetic inventory is the age that most closely approximates the number and type of the client's established consonants. For an analysis restricted only to intelligible words, a consonant is considered established when it occurs in at least two different words (the criterion used in the original studies). For an analysis of both intelligible and unintelligible words, a consonant is considered established when it occurs in at least three different words (the criterion used in the original study).

C. Error Patterns

1. **Appropriate Clients.** Analysis of error patterns is performed with clients in Stages 2 and 3 to help select short-term goals (see Chapter 4) and to determine the age level that best approximates the client's level of articulation and phonological development.

2. **Description.** Error patterns describe the client's accuracy in producing sound classes in the language of the client's community (see definition of relational analysis in Chapter 1, Section III). Error patterns encompass both what are traditionally called phonological processes and certain types of articulation errors (those affecting sound classes). As described in Chapter 2, the term error pattern is used in this book to avoid biasing the discussion to either an articulation or phonological perspective. A scale used to determine the

frequency with which an error pattern occurs in a client's speech is provided in Table 3-2. The categories in the scale are used to help select short-term treatment goals. The most likely candidates for short-term treatment goals are error patterns within the "present" category (see Chapter 4). A sample clinical form used to summarize the analysis of a client's error patterns is provided in Appendix 3L, and a sample clinical form showing when selected major error patterns are eliminated is presented in Appendix 3M.

D. Consonants and Consonants Clusters

1. **Appropriate Clients.** Analysis of consonants and consonant clusters is undertaken with clients in Stages 2 through 4 to help select treatment targets (see Chapter 4) and to establish the age that best approximates the level of the client's articulation and phonological development.

2. **Description.** Analysis of consonants and consonant clusters describes the client's ability to produce the individual consonants and consonant clusters in the language spoken in the client's community (see definition of relational analysis in Chapter 1, Section III). Analysis of consonants and consonant clusters is the longest established and still one of the most frequently used procedures in the care of clients with articulation and phonological disorders. A scale used to deter-

Table 3-2. Percentage and whole number criteria for disappearance of error patterns.

Categories	Percentages	Whole Numbers[a]	
		(5 Opportunities)	(10 Opportunities)
Highly frequent	75–100%	4/5–5/5	8/10–10/10
Frequent	50–74%	3/5	5/10–7/10
Present	25–49%	2/5	3/10–4/10
Disappearing	1–24%	1/5	1/10–2/10
Disappeared	0%	0/5	0/10

[a] Whole numbers refer to the number of different words. For example, 3/5 means the error pattern occurred in 3 out of 5 words.

mine the frequency with which a consonant and consonant cluster occurs in a client's speech is provided in Table 3–3. The categories in the scale are used to help select treatment targets. The most likely candidates for treatment targets are error patterns within the "emerging" category (see Chapter 4). The ages at which consonants and consonant clusters are typically acquired are listed in Tables 3–4 and 3–5, respectively (Smit, Hand, Frelinger, Bernthal, & Byrd, 1990). For the present purposes, to be considered acquired a sound needed to meet two criteria: (1) both males and females correctly produced the sound and (2) the percentage of subjects correctly producing the sound never dropped below 50% (for 50% criteria) or 75% (for 75% criteria) at any subsequent ages level. A sample clinical form used to analyze consonants and consonant clusters using a 50% acquisition criteria is provided in Appendix 3N.

E. Summary Comments

Age norms are extremely useful clinically but several factors limit their value.

   1. Normal Variation. The ages cited in age norms are averages. Some children fall above the average and others fall below.

Table 3–3. Percentage and whole number criteria for acquisition of consonants and consonant clusters.

Categories	Percentages	Whole Numbers[a]	
		(5 Opportunities)	(10 Opportunities)
Mastered	90–100%	5/5	9/10–10/10
Acquired	75–89 %	4/5	8/10
Present	50–74%	3/5	5/10–7/10
Emerging	10–49%	1/5 and 2/5	1/10–4/10
Rare	9%	1/5	—
Absent	0%	0/5	0/10

[a] Whole numbers refer to the number of different words. For example, 4/5 means the sound was produced correctly in 4 out of 5 words.

Table 3-4. Age of acquisition (50% to 75% correct) of American English consonants averaged across both word initial and word final positions.

Consonant	50%	75%	Consonant	50%	75%
m	<3;0	<3;0	ʃ	<3;0	3;6
n	<3;0	<3;0	v	3;6	4;6
ŋ	<3;0	<7;6[a]	θ	4;6	6;0
h	<3;0	<7;6	ɚ	4;6	5;6
w	<3;0	<3;0	s	3;6	5;0
j	<3;0	3;6	z	4;0	6;0
p	<3;0	<3;0	ʃ	3;6	5;0
t	<3;0	<3;0	tʃ	3;6	6;0
k	<3;0	<3;0	dʒ	3;6	4;6
b	<3;0	<3;0	r	3;6	6;0
d	<3;0	<3;0	l	3;6	6;0
g	<3;0	<3;0			

[a] Transcriber difficulties may have resulted in this sound being acquired at 7:6.

Source: Adapted from "The Iowa Articulation Norms Project and Its Nebraska Replication" by A. Smit, L. Hand, J. Frelinger, J. Bernthal, & A. Byrd (1990), *Journal of Speech and Hearing Disorders, 55,* 779–798.

Table 3-5. Age of acquisition (50% to 75% correct) of American English consonant clusters in word initial positions.

Cluster	50%	75%	Cluster	50%	75%
tw	3;0	3;6	pr	4;0	6;0
kw	3;0	3;6	br	3;6	6;0
sp	3;6	5;0	tr	5;0	5;6
st	3;6	5;0	dr	4;0	6;0
sk	3;6	5;0	kr	4;0	5;6
sm	3;6	5;0	gr	4;6	6;0
sn	3;6	5;6	fr	3;6	6;0
sw	3;6	5;6	θr	5;0	7;0
sl	4;6	7;0	skw	3;6	7;0
pl	3;6	5;6	spl	5;0	7;0
bl	3;6	5;0	spr	5;0	8;0
kl	4;0	5;6	str	5;0	8;0
gl	3;6	4;6	skr	5;0	8;0
fl	3;6	5;6			

Source: Adapted from "The Iowa Articulation Norms Project and Its Nebraska Replication" by A. Smit, L. Hand, J. Frelinger, J. Bernthal, & A. Byrd (1990), *Journal of Speech and Hearing Disorders, 55,* 779–798.

For example, a child might acquire a certain sound at 2 years, 4 months that age norms indicate should be acquired at 2 years. Is the child delayed or is this normal variation? The answer depends on the average variation (standard deviation) for acquiring the speech behavior being considered. If the average variation is, for example, 2 months, then a 4-month delay may signify an actual delay in articulation and phonological development. If, however, the average variation is 4 months, then the child's articulation and phonological development is within expected age limits. Unfortunately, information on average variation is often lacking, which makes it difficult to interpret results from clients with mild delays in articulation and phonological development.

2. **Ethnic and Class Biases.** Most age norms are derived from studies of Caucasian, middle class children. It is not known at present how useful this information is in interpreting assessment data from clients from other socioeconomic classes and ethnic and racial groups. Equally important, virtually no information exists on the priorities that members of non-Caucasian ethnic and racial groups assign to remediating various types of articulation and phonological disorders (Bleile & Wallach, 1992; Taylor & Peters-Johnson, 1986)

3. **Language Biases.** Almost all age norms are based on English-speaking children. At present, little is known about how children acquire speech in languages other than English. This gives our field a narrow, ethnocentric view of articulation and phonological development. Additionally, this lack of normative information about other languages makes it almost impossible to evaluate the speech of non-English-speaking clients.

V. BETTER ABILITIES

Better abilities are the client's more advanced articulation and phonological abilities. Better abilities are a primary means used to select treatment targets (see Chapter 4). Several procedures help to identify the client's better abilities: stimulability testing, key environments, key words, and phonetic placement and shaping.

A. Stimulability Testing

1. **Appropriate Clients.** Stimulability testing is performed rou-

tinely with clients in Stages 2 through 4 to help select treatment targets (see Chapter 4).

2. **Description.** Stimulability is the ability to say a treatment target correctly during delayed or immediate imitation. A client who pronounces [k] correctly during imitation, for example, is considered stimulable for [k]. The logic behind stimulability testing is that sounds that can be produced correctly during imitation are easier for clients to acquire than treatment targets that cannot be imitated. Many times, hypotheses about stimulability are tested while collecting the speech sample. A clinician, for example, might ask the client to name pictures, and then ask the client to imitate words that the client pronounced incorrectly. Hypotheses about stimulability can also be tested using the same procedure during the course of eliciting speech through word probes for sounds and error patterns. Another option to test for stimulability is to present the client a word list specially developed for this purpose. Such a word list is provided in Appendix 3O.

B. Key Environments

1. **Appropriate Clients.** Analysis of key environments is performed with clients in Stages 2 through 4 to help select treatment targets (see Chapter 4).

2. **Description.** A key environment is a phonetic environment in which the client is able to successfully produce a sound or class of sounds. Key environments often are syllable and word positions, but may also include the presence of other sounds. An example of a word (and syllable) key environment is a client who can produce velar stops only at the ends of words. An example of a key environment that includes the presence of another sound is a client who can produce a labial consonant only at the beginning of a word if the word also ends in a labial consonant, or a client who can produce [t] only when followed by a front vowel in the same syllable. Key environments vary by client, so that, for example, word-final position may be a key environment for velar stops for one client, but not for another. The speech of yet other clients may not contain any key environments, containing, instead, sounds that are produced with some success across several environments.

To discover whether a key environment exists for a sound, the clinician should ask him- or herself, "Is there any phonetic environment in which the client is successful in producing the sound?" Key environments are often first discovered during the collection of the initial speech sample. Typically, hypotheses about possible key environments are tested using word probes such as those presented in Chapter 2. More uncommon key environments are tested using word probes developed by the clinician (Bleile, 1991b).

Although individual differences in key environments are extensive, the following is a list of "first bets" for the phonetic contexts in which to look for key environments (for a similar list of key environments in which to establish sounds see Table 4–4):

The beginning of words is the most common key environment for consonants.

Between vowels is sometimes a key environment for voiced consonants, especially voiced fricatives.

The ends of syllables and words are sometimes key environments for voiceless consonants.

The ends of syllables and words are sometimes key environments for velar consonants. Another key environment for velar stops may be before back vowels in the same syllable, as in "go."

The beginnings of syllables and words before a front vowel are sometimes key environments for alveolar consonants, as in "tea."

C. Key Words

1. **Appropriate Clients.** Analysis of key words is performed with clients from Stage 2 through Stage 4 to help select treatment targets (see Chapter 4).

2. **Description.** Key words occur when a client's success in producing a sound is limited to a few specific words. Many times key words are of special importance to the client. During the years when the "Star Wars" movies were at the height of

their popularity, for example, the name of the movies' villain, Darth Vader, was a key word for [v] for many children. Names of favorite friends and characters in television series are also "first bets" when trying to find key words. Key words need not be "special" to the client, and, in fact, any word can be a key word. Key words are typically discovered while collecting the initial speech sample or performing hypothesis testing. Because key words are often useful in treatment, the clinician should circle key words as they are discovered or in other some manner indicate that a key word exists.

D. Phonetic Placement and Shaping

1. **Appropriate Clients.** Brief trials using phonetic placement and shaping are performed with more mature and cognitively advanced clients in Stage 3 and clients in Stage 4 to help select treatment targets (see Chapter 4).

2. **Description.** Phonetic placement and shaping techniques physically direct a client to produce a sound. A phonetic placement technique for [t], for example, might involve directing the client to touch his or her tongue tip to the alveolar ridge. The logic behind including brief trials of phonetic placement and shaping techniques in the assessment is to determine if they provide the client a means to produce a difficult sound. A relatively complete description of phonetic placement and shaping techniques is presented in Appendix 5C.

E. Summary Comments

When analyzing a client's speech, it is equally (or more) important to determine the client's areas of strength as it is to establish the client's deficit areas. The analysis of better abilities is undertaken to identify the client's more advanced articulation and phonological skills. The information gained from these analyses is often useful in selecting treatment targets.

The primary types of analyses of better abilities involve stimulability, key environments, key words, and phonetic placement and shaping. A natural question raised by stimulability testing is whether a client who is stimulable for a treatment target would make progress even if treatment was not provided. Research on this question is equivocal (Diedrich, 1983; Madison, 1979; Powell, Elbert, & Dinnsen, 1991). More studies are needed before the predictive value of stimulability is known. Until then, stimulability provides a quick method for choosing treatment targets that are likely to meet with success. Key environments and key words provide important means for selecting treatment targets for clients in Stages 2 through 4. Brief trials using phonetic placement and shaping techniques provide useful methods to determine if selected clients in Stage 3 and clients in Stage 4 might benefit from use of these techniques during treatment.

VI. RELATED ANALYSES

Several analyses are performed in conjunction with the above assessments. Some analyses are performed with virtually all clients; others are restricted to clients in selected clinical populations. Because the analyses described in this section are united only by their "related" status, summary comments are provided after each subheading rather than at the end of the section.

A. Adjusted Age

1. **Appropriate Clients.** Adjusted age is determined for infants and toddlers born prematurely to determine the client's potential for articulation and phonological development.

2. **Description.** Adjusted age is the client's chronological age adjusted for prematurity. Adjusted age is calculated for clients 24 months or younger who were born prematurely to establish the client's best potential for articulation and phonological development. For example, a client with a chronological age of 22 months and an adjusted age of 20 months is expected to have the articulation and phonological skills of a child 20 months of age, not a child 22 months of age. A sample clinical form used to determine adjusted age is provided in Appendix 3P.

3. **Summary Comments.** Adjusted age is not calculated for clients older than 24 months, because by that age children born prematurely are thought to have "caught up" in development.

B. Developmental Age

1. **Appropriate Clients.** Developmental age is calculated for clients with intellectual or cognitive impairments to establish the client's potential for articulation and phonological development.

2. **Description.** Developmental age (also called mental age) is the age that most closely corresponds to the client's level of cognitive development. Developmental age is calculated for clients with intellectual or cognitive impairments to determine the client's potential for articulation and phonological development. For example, a client whose chronological age is 9 years, but whose developmental age is 6 years, is expected to have the articulation and phonological development commensurate to a child 6 years of age. A sample clinical form used to determine developmental age is provided in Appendix 3Q.

3. **Summary Comments.** Developmental age is best calculated using a verbal intelligence quotient (verbal IQ). In clinical practice, the standard score from the *Peabody Picture Vocabulary Test — Revised* (PPVT-R) (Dunn & Dunn, 1981) is sometimes used to determine developmental age, because PPVT-R scores are positively correlated with verbal intelligence. It should be noted, however, that the correlation between a client's PPVT-R score and his or her verbal intelligence is not always reliable (Dunn & Dunn, 1981); therefore, determination of a person's verbal intelligence based on a PPVT-R score must be made with caution. With younger clients, the level of the client's language reception abilities is often used to approximate developmental age.

C. Dialect

1. **Appropriate Clients.** The influence of dialect is identified in all appropriate clients in Stages 2 through 4 to differentiate dialect from speech characteristics that signify a possible articulation and phonological disorder.

Dialect Reduction

Techniques used to treat articulation and phonological disorders can also be used to reduce dialect. I have

some concern about providing dialect reduction, because such treatment may confirm the impression of
some persons (including the client) that dialect is a type
of disorder. Nonetheless, I occasionally provide this
clinical service, because in my opinion the client's right
to clinical care for what he or she perceives to be a problem outweighs other considerations. I accompany treatment for dialect reduction with an educational program
on the nature of dialects.

2. **Description.** Dialect is a variation in language resulting from
the influence of a region, social group, racial group, or ethnic group. Sample clinical forms used to help identify possible dialect characteristics in two major ethnic dialects, Black
English Vernacular (BEV) and Hawaiian Island Creole
(HC), are provided in Appendixes 3R and 3S, respectively.

3. **Summary Comments.** Dialects are a natural part of language, and dialect characteristics need to be identified in all
appropriate clients so that they will not be diagnosed as articulation and phonological disorders.

Limited English Proficiency

Discussion of speakers with limited English proficiency
lies beyond the scope of this book. The reader is referred to Cheng (1987) and Goldstein (in press) for excellent discussions of assessing speech and language in
Asian and Spanish populations, respectively.

D. Acquisition Strategies

1. **Appropriate Clients.** Analysis of acquisition strategies is
undertaken with clients in Stage 2 and less advanced clients
in Stage 3 to identify the possible influence of learning style
on assessment and treatment.

2. **Description.** Acquisition strategies represent approaches to learning how to speak. The hallmarks of various acquisition strategies are listed in Table 3–6. Although acquisition strategies are often readily identifiable by clinicians who are attuned to their possible presence, in-depth analyses of acquisition strategies can be extremely time consuming and typically are not performed in clinical settings. Differing from other sections in this chapter, the following discussion is intended to facilitate identification rather than describe specific analytic procedures. The interested reader is referred to the references cited below for procedures used to analyze acquisition strategies.

   a. **Regressions.** Regressions are temporary losses of articulation and phonological abilities. Some regressions involve a loss in phonetic accuracy in a single word, whereas others may alter previously "correct" stress patterns, syllable shapes, or sound classes (Bleile & Tomblin, 1991; Menn, 1976). Regressions appear to arise as the client generalizes and overgeneralizes "regular ways to say words." Similar to morphological overgeneralization (e.g., when a

Table 3–6. Major articulation and phonological acquisition strategies.

Strategies	Hallmark
Regressions	The client temporarily loses a speech ability. A temporary regression may last from days to months.
Favorite sounds	The client uses a sound (sometimes an unusual one, such as syllabic [s]) in place of many other sounds.
Selectivity	The client "picks and chooses" words that contain sounds and sound sequences that he or she already produces.
Word recipes	The client's words are organized into a few sound patterns.
Word-based leaning	The client's pronunciation of a sound varies depending on the word in which it occurs.
Gestalt learning	The client knows "the tune before the words."

preschooler overgeneralizes the past tense marker to say, "I goed home"), articulation and phonological regressions actually represent progress in development. Temporary regressions lasting from days to months are relatively common. Unless the regressions are concomitant with changes in neurological status, their presence is not cause for concern and, indeed, may signify important developmental advances.

b. **Favorite Sounds.** Favorite sounds are consonants and vowels that occur with high frequency in the client's speech. A favorite sound, for example, might be an [s] that the client uses to pronounce all words that in the adult language begin with fricatives, stops, or affricates (Ferguson & Macken, 1983). Although having favorite sounds is not a disability, extensive use of favorite sounds may result in increased homonomy and may signify difficulty in acquiring a repertoire of diverse speech sounds. In other clinical situations, however, the clinician may choose to facilitate the acquisition of words that contain the client's favorite sounds.

c. **Selectivity.** Selectivity is the ability some clients demonstrate to "pick and choose" the sounds and sound sequences they will attempt to pronounce. In general, children appear to choose words that contain sounds already in their expressive vocabularies (Schwartz, 1988; Schwartz & Leonard, 1982). A client, for example, may have an expressive vocabulary containing words beginning with [t] and [k] and only be willing to attempt to pronounce new words that begin with the same sounds. Selectivity is sometimes useful in selecting treatment targets, because clients who engage in selectivity may be more likely to attempt words with familiar sounds and sound sequences (see Chapter 4).

d. **Word Recipes.** Word recipes are simple formulas that some clients appear to use to simplify the task of speaking. The term word recipes is intended to convey that some clients, like some inexperienced cooks, use very few recipes over and over again (Menn, 1976; Waterson, 1971). A client, for example, might have two-word recipes that are used to pronounce almost all words in his or her expressive vocabulary. One word recipe might be, "All words that are monosyllables in the adult language are pronounced as CV and the consonant is [d]," and the other word recipe might be, "All words that are multisyllabic in the adult language are pronounced CVCV, and both consonants are identical in place of production." Clients whose acquisition strategies include word recipes may find it easier to acquire words that follow their word recipes. More negatively, the speech of clients who follow this strategy is often highly unintelligible, because these clients only have a few means to pronounce a large number of sounds and syllables.

e. Homonyms. Homonyms are words that sound alike but have different meanings. Some clients appear unbothered by the degree of homonomy in their speech; others appear to produce unusual pronunciations to avoid having too many homonyms (Ingram, 1975). A client's degree of homonomy is determined simply by dividing the number of different homonyms in the client's expressive vocabulary by the total number of words. Reduction in homophonyms is a possible short-term treatment goal (see Chapter 1).

f. Word-based Learning. Word-based learning uses words to organize the articulation and phonological systems. The hallmark of word-based learning is that how a client pronounces a sound depends on the word in which it occurs (Ferguson & Farwell, 1975). For example, a word beginning with [p] in the adult language may be pronounced by the client as [b] in one word, as [t] in another word, and as [p] or [s] in other words. Word-based sound systems disappear as the client discovers "regular ways to say words," which typically occurs as the child's expressive vocabulary grows to contain 50 or more words. The change from word-based learning to rule-based learning may be one source of articulation and phonological regressions. For example, the client in the above example might generalize [t] to all words that begin with [p] in the adult language, resulting in a temporary regression in words that previously had been pronounced with an initial [p]. Although word-based learning is not a form of disability, persistent use of this acquisition strategy results in extensive variability in the production of sounds. Reduction in variability is a possible treatment goal in selected clients (see Chapter 4).

g. **Gestalt learning.** Gestalt learning typically involves "learning the tune before the words" (Peters, 1977, 1983). Clients prone to gestalt learning may accurately produce sentence intonation (the tune), although the pronunciation of words within the sentence may be poor. Sometimes clients who pronounce the intonation of sentences better than the sounds in the sentence are said to be speaking "jargon." Clients speaking "jargon" are often extremely difficult to understand, because the sounds within the words are highly inaccurate.

3. **Summary Comments.** The existence of acquisition strategies serves to remind us that clients are actively engaged in the process of articulation and phonological development. Rather than proceeding in a straight line, articulation and phonological acquisition zigzags and sometimes even regresses as the client generalizes and overgeneralizes rules. Some clients may have favorite sounds or be very selective in the words they will attempt to say; others may develop simple "word recipes" which they use to pronounce almost all words. Homonomy sometimes serves as an acquisition strategy. Some clients seem to favor increased homonomy, while others seem to develop ways to pronounce words to avoid homonyms. Many clients follow a word-based strategy in which how a sound is pronounced depends on the word in which it occurs. Finally, some clients appear to focus less on the pronunciation of words and more on the intonation patterns in which words occur.

APPENDIX 3A
4-Point Clinical Judgment
Scale of Severity

A. Instruction

Ask one or more speech-language clinicians familiar with the client's speech to independently mark the number on the assessment scale below that, in their professional judgment, best describes the client's severity of articulation and phonological involvement. If more than one judge is used, add the judges' scores and divide the total by the number of judges to obtain an average score. An average score of between 3 and 4 is commonly needed to receive articulation and phonological services, although a less stringent criterion is possible with clients who have risk factors for future articulation and phonological development.

B. Assessment Scale

☐ 1 No disorder

☐ 2 Mild disorder

☐ 3 Moderate disorder

☐ 4 Severe disorder

APPENDIX 3B
3-Point Clinical Judgment
Scale of Severity

A. Instructions

Ask one or more speech-language clinicians familiar with the client to independently check the statements on the assessment scale below that in their professional judgment describe the client's speech. Each statement is rated 1 or 0. Typically, an average score of 1 or more is needed to justify articulation and phonological services.

B. Assessment Scale

☐ The client's speech has or in the future is likely to have an adverse affect on his or her social development and educational progress.

☐ The client's speech calls attention to itself.

☐ The client's speech is delayed relative to developmental age norms.

APPENDIX 3C
Percentage of Consonants Correct (PCC)

A. Instructions

Calculate the client's PCC percentage using the procedures described below and on the following pages. The level of severity needed to obtain articulation and phonological services varies by clinical setting. A score of 50–65% or less is recommended for most client populations. A less stringent criterion — 65% or higher — is recommended for clients at risk for future articulation and phonological difficulties.

B. Step 1: Collect Data and Identify Utterances

The following data collection procedures are used:

Obtain a continuous speech sample of between 50 to 100 utterances.

Determine the meaning of the utterances.

Identify any dialect characteristics (example: "aks" or "ask" in Black English Vernacular).

Identify casual speech pronunciations (example: "Cheat yet?" for "Did you eat yet?").

Identify allophones (example: [ɾ] for [t] in "butter").

C. Step 2: Exclusion Criteria

Exclude the following data from analysis:

Exclude all unintelligible and partially intelligible utterances.

Exclude vowels (including [ɚ]).

Do not count the addition of consonants in front of vowels (example: "hit" for "it") because the target is a vowel.

Exclude consonants in the third or more repetition of the same word, if the pronunciation does not change (example: count only the first two instances of [b] in three or more repetitions of "bee" [bi bi bi]).

Exclude beyond the second consonant in successive utterances with the same pronunciation, but score all consonants if the pronunciation changes.

D. Step 3: Identify Errors in the Remaining Data

Follow these criteria to identify consonant errors:

Score dialect, casual speech, and allophones based on the consonant the client intended (example: "aks" for "ask" is correct in BEV, but "ats" is incorrect).

Score a consonant as incorrect if in doubt about whether it is correct or incorrect.

Score consonant deletions as incorrect (example: "be" for "bed).

Score consonant substitutions as incorrect (example: "bee" for "pea").

Score partial voicing of initial consonants as incorrect.

Score distortions (no matter how mild) as incorrect.

Score additions of a sound to consonant as incorrect (example: "mits" for "miss")

Score initial [h] and [n/ŋ] substitutions in stressed syllables as incorrect, but not in unstressed syllables (example: "swin" for "swing" is incorrect, but "jumpin" for "jumping" is correct).

E. Step 4: Calculate PCC

Perform the following calculation to determine PCC:

1. Formula

$$\frac{\text{total number of correct consonants}}{\text{total number of intended consonants}} \times 100 = \text{PCC}$$

2. Example

$$\frac{70 \text{ consonants correct}}{100 \text{ consonants attempted}} \times 100 = 70\%$$

F. Step 5: Determine level of Severity

Indicate the client's level of severity using the following scale:

85%	= Normal development	☐
65–85%	= Mild to moderate disorder	☐
50–65%	= Moderate to severe disorder	☐
<50%	= Severe disorder	☐

APPENDIX 3D
Articulation Competence Index (ACI)

A. Instructions

Calculate the client's ACI using the procedures described below and on the following pages. A score of 70% or higher suggests the need for articulation and phonological services. A lower score might indicate the need for services if the client was judged at risk for future articulation and phonological difficulties.

B. Step 1: Collect Data

Follow the data collection procedures as for the PCC (Appendix 3C).

C. Step 2: Exclude Nonclinical Distortions from Analysis

Exclude all nonclinical distortions due to regional, ethnic, or socioeconomic influence.

D. Step 3: Identify Clinical Distortions

The following are scored as clinical distortions:

[l] or [r] with lip rounding

[l] or [r] made in the velar position

[r] and r-colored vowels produced as vowels

Lateralized sibilant fricatives or affricates

Lisped sibilant fricatives or affricates

Weakly produced consonants

Imprecise consonants and vowels

Failure to maintain oral/nasal contrasts (nasal emissions, denasalized nasal consonants, nasalized oral consonants, and nasalized vowels and diphthongs)

Notable failure to maintain appropriate voicing (nonaspiration of prevocalic voiceless stops, voicing of voiceless obstruents, and partial devoicing of voiced obstruents)

E. Step 4: Calculate Percentage of Consonants Correct (PCC)

Calculate the PCC using the following formula.

1. Formula

$$\frac{\text{total number of correct consonants}}{\text{total number of intended consonants}} \times 100 = \text{PCC}$$

2. Example

$$\frac{70 \text{ consonants correct}}{100 \text{ consonants attempted}} \times 100 = 70\%$$

F. Step 5: Calculate Relative Distortion Index (RDI):

Calculate RDI using the following formula:

1. Formula

$$\frac{\text{total number of distortion errors}}{\text{total number of speech errors}} \times = \text{RDI}$$

2. Example

$$\frac{60 \text{ distortions}}{70 \text{ speech errors}} \times = 85.71\% \ (86\%)$$

G. Step 6: Calculated ACI:

Calculate ACI using the following formula:

1. Formula

$$\frac{\text{PCC} + \text{RDI}}{2} \times \text{ACI}$$

2. Example

$$\frac{70 + 86}{2} = 78\%$$

APPENDIX 3E
Percentage of Development

A. Instructions

Determine the age equivalent corresponding to the client's articulation and phonological development using the formula described below. Next, divide the age equivalent score (in months) by the client's age (in months). Use adjusted age rather than chronological age with clients 24 months or younger who were born prematurely. The specific percentage needed to qualify for articulation and phonological services varies by state. New Jersey, for example, uses a 33% delay as the criteria for developmental services.

1. Formula

$$\frac{\text{developmental age in months}}{\text{chronological age in months}} = \text{percentage of delay}$$

2. Example

$$\frac{24 \text{ months}}{36 \text{ months}} = 33\% \text{ delay in development}$$

APPENDIX 3F
3-Point Clinical Judgment Scale
of Intelligibility

A. Instructions

Ask one or more speech-language clinicians familiar with the client to place a check mark next to the statements on the assessment scales below that in their professional judgment describe the client's intelligibility during conversation. If more than one judge is used, add the judges' scores and divide the total by the number of judges. The "score" needed to obtain service for a possible articulation and phonological disorder varies by setting and age of the client.

B. Assessment Scale

☐   1   Readily intelligible

☐   2   Intelligible if topic is known

☐   3   Unintelligible even with careful listening

APPENDIX 3G
5-Point Clinical Judgment Scale
of Intelligibility

A. Instructions

Ask one or more speech-language clinicians familiar with the client to place a check mark next to the statements on the assessment scales below that in their professional judgment describe the client's intelligibility during conversation. If more than one judge is used, add the scores and divide the total by the number of judges to obtain an average score. The "score" needed to obtain service for a possible articulation and phonological disorder varies by setting and age of the client.

B. Assessment Scale

☐   1   Completely intelligible

☐   2   Mostly intelligible

☐   3   Somewhat intelligible

☐   4   Mostly unintelligible

☐   5   Completely unintelligible

APPENDIX 3H
Percentage of Occurrence of English Consonants

A. Instructions

Identify the client's consonant errors and place a check mark next to consonants listed on the assessment scale that the client produces incorrectly. The list is arranged in descending order from greatest to least frequent in occurrence.

B. Assessment Scale[a]

Percentage of Occurrence of English Consonants

Consonant	Rank	Percentage	Consonant	Rank	Percentage
t _____	1	13.7	p _____	13	3.9
n _____	2	11.7	b _____	14	3.5
s _____	3	7.1	z _____	15	3.0
k _____	4	6.0	ŋ _____	16	2.5
d _____	5	5.8	f _____	17	2.4
m _____	6	5.6	j _____	18	2.2
l _____	7	5.6	ʃ _____	19	1.5
r _____	8	5.2	v _____	20	1.2
w _____	9	4.8	θ _____	21	0.9
h _____	10	4.2	tʃ _____	22	0.7
ð _____	11	4.1	tʒ _____	23	0.6
g _____	12	4.1	ʒ _____	24	0.0

---

[a] The data source for this assessment scale is Shriberg and Kwiatkowski (1983).

APPENDIX 31
Effect of Error Patterns
on Intelligibility

A. Instructions

Identify the client's error patterns and place a check mark next to any patterns on the assessment form on the scale below that occur in the client's speech. The list of error patterns is arranged in descending order from most to least effect on intelligibility.

B. Assessment Scale[1]

Beginning of Word

Most to least effect:

Fronting _____

Gliding _____

Initial voicing _____

Stopping _____

Cluster reduction _____

End of Word

Most to least effect:

Final Consonant Deletion _____

Fronting _____

Word Final Devoicing _____

---

[1] The data source for this assessment scale is Leinonen-Davies (1988).

APPENDIX 3J
Prespeech Vocalizations[1]

A. Instructions

Obtain a speech sample following the procedures described in Chapter Two. Place check marks next to the age levels corresponding to the client's vocalizations on the assessment scale below. The age equivalent of the client's vocal development is the most advanced age at which an established vocalization occurs.

B. Assessment Scale[1]

Prespeech Vocalization

Present	Approximate Age	Milestones
___ ___ ___	0–6 weeks	Crying, fussing, vegetative sounds
___ ___ ___	2–3 months	Begins to produce cooing behaviors
___ ___ ___	2–4 months	Begins to produce pleasure sounds such as "mmmm"
___ ___ ___	3–4 months	Cooing behavior is well established, babbling behavior (repetition or consonants and vowels) begins to appear
___ ___ ___	4 months	Produces some intonation during sound making and may engage in vocal play when playing with toys; vocalizations begin to be dominated by sounds produced at the front of the mouth, including raspberries and trills
___ ___ ___	7–8 months	Produces reduplicated babbling (repetition of same syllable)
___ ___ ___	10 months	Produces nonreduplicative babbling (changes of consonants and vowels within syllables)

---

[1] The data source for this appendix is Stark (1980). The checklist was adapted from J. Vannucci (1994).

APPENDIX 3K
Phonetic Inventories[1]

A. Instructions

Obtain a speech sample following the procedures described in Chapter 2. Tally the client's consonants using the forms on the following pages, placing a hash mark above each consonant the client produces. For example, if the client says [bi], [bu], and [ip], place two hash marks above [b] on the word-initial form and one hash mark above [p] on the word-final form. Circle consonants that the client produces in two or more different words (if analyzing only intelligible speech) or three or more different words (if analyzing both unintelligible and intelligible speech). Next, compare the client's consonant development to the inventories listed in either Phonetic Inventories (Intelligible Speech) or Phonetic Inventories (Intelligible and Unintelligible Speech). Look for the closest match between the client's consonant inventory and that listed on the phonetic inventory forms, expecting that your client's consonant inventory is not likely to exactly match the number and types of consonants shown on the phonetic inventory forms.

---

[1] The data sources for this appendix are Stoel-Gammon (1985), Dyson (1988), and Robb and Bleile (in press).

B. Sample Form for Determining Phonetic Inventories in Word-Initial Position

Manner of Production	Place of Production						
	Bilabial	Labiodental	Interdental	Alveolar	Postalveolar	Palatal	Velar	Glottal
Oral Stop	p b			t d			k g	
Fricative		f v	ɵ ð	s z	ʃ			
Affricate					tʃ dʒ			
Nasal Stop	m			n				
Liquid								
Central				r				
Lateral				l				
Glide	w					j		h

164

C. Sample Form for Determining Phonetic Inventories in Word-Final Position

Manner of Production	Place of Production							
	Bilabial	Labiodental	Interdental	Alveolar	Postalveolar	Palatal	Velar	Glottal
Oral Stop	p b			t d			k g	
Fricative		f v	θ ð	s z	ʃ ʒ			
Affricate					tʃ dʒ			
Nasal Stop	m			n			ŋ	
Liquid								
Central				r				
Lateral				l				

D. Phonetic Inventories (Intelligible Speech)

Highest Level	Age (in mos)	Position	Number of Consonants	Typical Consonants
_____	15	Initial	3	b d h
_____		Final	none	ø
_____	18	Initial	6	b d m n h w
_____		Final	1	t
_____	24	Initial	9	b d g t k m n h w f s
_____		Final	6	p t k n r s
_____	29	Initial	14	b d g p t k m n h w j f s l
_____		Final	11	d p t k m n ŋ f s ʃ tʃ

E. Phonetic Inventories (Intelligible and Unintelligible Speech)

Highest Level	Age (in mos)	Position	Number of Consonants	Typical Consonants
_____	12	Initial	5	b d h g m h
_____		Final	1	m
_____	18	Initial	6	b d m n h w
_____		Final	2	t s
_____	24	Initial	10	b d p t k m n h s w
_____		Final	4	t k n s

APPENDIX 3L
Summary Form for Error Probe Analysis

A. Instructions

Obtain a speech sample during the initial assessment using either standardized or nonstandardized procedures. Next, perform error probes for the error patterns you consider most likely to be treatment targets, postponing consideration of more minor and infrequent error patterns. Use either the error probe forms themselves or, if desired, the form below to tabulate the results of the error probe analysis. The following example shows how the form is used to summarize the error probe for Fronting and Lisping. Whole numbers refer to the number of different words in which the error pattern occurred. For example, 8/10 means the error pattern occurred in 8 of 10 words.

B. Example

Error Patterns	Occurrence	Stimulability
Fronting	8/10	Yes (words: key, go)
Lisping	10/10	No

C. Summary Form for Error Probe Analysis

Error Patterns	Occurrence	Stimulability
Changes in Place of Production		
Fronting***	_____	_____
Lisping***	_____	_____
Velar Assimilation***	_____	_____
Labial Assimilation***	_____	_____
Backing	_____	_____
Glottal Replacement	_____	_____

continued

Summary Form (continued)

Error Patterns	Occurrence	Stimulability
Changes in Manner of Production		
Stopping***	_____	_____
Gliding***	_____	_____
Lateralization***	_____	_____
Affrication	_____	_____
Nasalization	_____	_____
Densalization	_____	_____
Changes in the Beginning of Syllables or Words		
Prevocalic Voicing***	_____	_____
Initial Consonant Deletion	_____	_____
Changes at the End of Syllables or Words		
Final Consonant Devoicing***		_____
Final Consonant Deletion***	_____	_____
Changes in Syllables		
Reduplication***	_____	_____
Syllable Deletion***	_____	_____
Changes in Consonant Clusters		
Cluster Reduction***	_____	_____
Epenthesis***	_____	_____
Sound Reversals		
Metathesis	_____	_____
Changes in Vowels and Syllabic Consonants		
Vowel Neutralization***	_____	_____
Vocalization***	_____	_____

APPENDIX 3M
Typical Ages at Which Selected Major
Error Patterns Disappear

A. Instructions

Obtain a speech sample using either error probes (Appendix 2B) or through some other method. Next, identify the error patterns on the assessment scale on the next page that are expected to have disappeared below the client's chronological or developmental age.

B. Typical Ages at which Selected Major Error Patterns Disappear[1]

Disappear Before 3;0

_____ Prevocalic Voicing

_____ Velar Assimilation

_____ Labial Assimilation

_____ Reduplication

_____ Final Consonant Deletion

_____ Fronting

_____ Syllable Deletion

Disappear After 3;0

_____ Epenthesis

_____ Gliding

_____ Cluster Reduction

_____ Final Consonant Devoicing

_____ Stopping

---

[1] The data source for this appendix is Stoel-Gammon and Dunn (1985).

APPENDIX 3N
Acquisition of American English
Consonants and Consonant Clusters[1]

A. Instructions

Obtain a speech sample following either the standardized or non-standardized procedures described in Chapter 2. Place a check mark next to consonants and consonant clusters that the client produces correctly. If using the information for children under 3 years old, consonants must be produced correctly in at least two of three word positions (initial, medial, final). If using the information for older children, consonants must be produced correctly in both word-initial and word-final position and consonant clusters must be produced correctly in word-initial position.

B. Acquisition of American English Consonants

Consonant	Age	Consonant	Age
m	<2;0 ___	f	<3;0 ___
n	<2;0 ___	v	3;6 ___
ŋ	2;0 ___	θ	4;6 ___
h	<2;0 ___	ð	4;6 ___
w	<2;0 ___	s	3;6 ___
j	<3;0 ___	z	4;0 ___
p	<2;0 ___	ʃ	3;6 ___
t	2;0 ___	tʃ	3;6 ___
k	2;0 ___	dʒ	3;6 ___
b	<2;0 ___	r	3;6 ___
d	2;0 ___	l	3;6 ___
g	2;0 ___		

[1] The data sources for this appendix are Sander (1972) and Smit, Hand, Frelinger, Bernthal, & Byrd (1990). Data from Sander (1972) are for children under 3 years of age. Data from Smit et al. (1990) met two criteria: (1) at least 50% of both males and females correctly produced the sound in word initial and word final positions (consonants) or word initial position (consonant clusters), and (2) the percentage of subjects correctly producing the sound at subsequent age levels never dropped below 50%.

C. Acquisition of American English Consonant Clusters

Cluster	Age		Cluster	Age
tw	3;0 ____		pr	4;0 ____
kw	3;0 ____		br	3;6 ____
sp	3;6 ____		tr	5;0 ____
st	3;6 ____		dr	4;0 ____
sk	3;6 ____		kr	4;0 ____
sm	3;6 ____		gr	4;6 ____
sn	3;6 ____		fr	3;6 ____
sw	3;6 ____		θr	5;0 ____
sl	4;6 ____		skw	3;6 ____
pl	3;6 ____		spl	5;0 ____
bl	3;6 ____		spr	5;0 ____
kl	4;0 ____		str	5;0 ____
gl	3;6 ____		skr	5;0 ____
fl	3;6 ____			

APPENDIX 3O
Stimulability

A. Instructions

Determine which sounds you wish to test, and then ask the client to imitate the appropriate words, place a check mark next to consonants and consonant clusters for which the client is stimulable. The assessment scale in this appendix is organized according to the typical age of acquisition of consonants and consonant clusters. Stimulability is tested in three word positions (initial, medial, and final) for sounds acquired under 3 years of age. Consonants acquired at 3 years or older are tested in two word positions (initial and final). Consonant clusters are tested in word-initial position. Readers wishing to test stimulability in a greater number of word positions are referred to Appendix 2B for a word list not organized according to age of acquisition.

B. Stimulability Assessment Scale[1]

<2;0

[w]

#	S__S
wind	flower
wet	tower
win	shower

[m]

#	S__S	__#
moon	mama	game
mop	gummy	boom
mud	hammer	swim

[h]

#
home
hat
help

[n]

#	S__S	__#
nice	honey	spoon
new	rainy	fun
knife	tiny	pan

continued

---

[1] The data sources for this appendix are Sander (1972) and Smit, Hand, Frelinger, Bernthal, & Byrd (1990). Data from Sander (1972) are for children under 3 years of age. The consonants were produced correctly in 2 of 3 word positions (initial, medial, and final). Data from Smit et al. (1990) met two criteria: (1) at least 50% of both males and females correctly produced the sound in word-initial and word-final positions (consonants) or word-initial position (consonant clusters), and (2) the percentage of subjects correctly producing the sound at subsequent age levels never dropped below 50%. The Smit et al. data does not contain information for [ɹ] consonant clusters.

173

<2;0 *(continued)*

[p]

# ___		S ___ S		___ #	
pan	___	puppy	___	ape	___
pot	___	diaper	___	map	___
pie	___	sleepy	___	hop	___

[b]

# ___		S ___ S		___ #	
bee	___	baby	___	crab	___
bat	___	hobby	___	bib	___
book	___	tuba	___	tub	___

[ŋ]

___ #		S ___ S	
sing	___	singing	___
king	___	winging	___
hang	___	hanger	___

2;0

[d]

# ___		S ___ S		___ #	
dive	___	soda	___	kid	___
dog	___	daddy	___	mud	___
doll	___	birdie	___	bed	___

[t]

# ___		S ___ S		___ #	
tea	___	twenty	___	ate	___
tag	___	water	___	bat	___
toe	___	waiter	___	boat	___

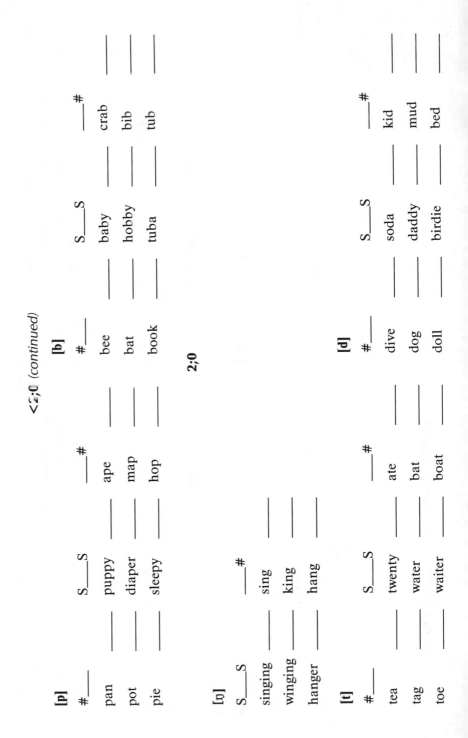

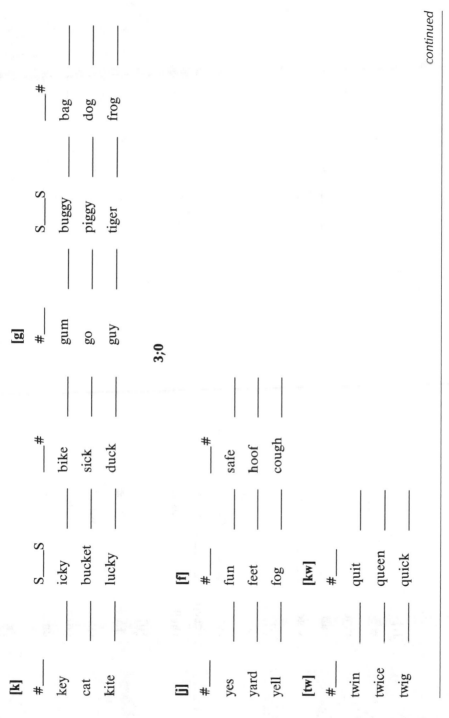

[k]

# __	S __ S	__ #
key	icky	bike
cat	bucket	sick
kite	lucky	duck

[g]

# __	S __ S	__ #
gum	buggy	bag
go	piggy	dog
guy	tiger	frog

3;0

[f]

# __	__ #
fun	safe
feet	hoof
fog	cough

[j]

__
yes
yard
yell

[kw]

__
quit
queen
quick

[tw]

__
twin
twice
twig

continued

175

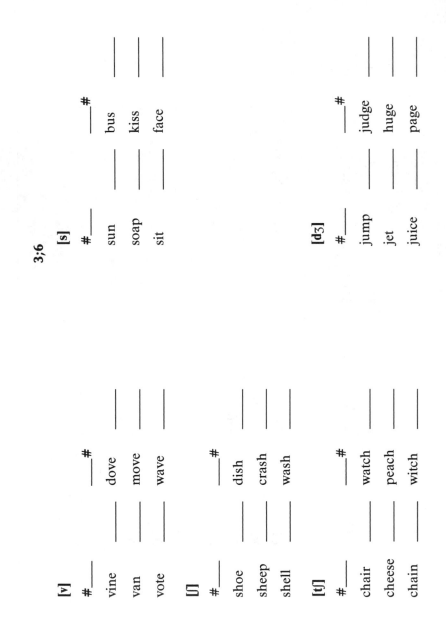

3;6

[v]

# ___	# ___
vine ___	dove ___
van ___	move ___
vote ___	wave ___

[ʃ]

# ___	# ___
shoe ___	dish ___
sheep ___	crash ___
shell ___	wash ___

[tʃ]

# ___	# ___
chair ___	watch ___
cheese ___	peach ___
chain ___	witch ___

[s]

# ___	# ___
sun ___	bus ___
soap ___	kiss ___
sit ___	face ___

[dʒ]

# ___	# ___
jump ___	judge ___
jet ___	huge ___
juice ___	page ___

[l]

# ___		___ #	
light	___	ball	___
laugh	___	fall	___
left	___	eel	___

[r]

# ___		___ #	
rain	___	car	___
row	___	air	___
root	___	chair	___

[sp]

# ___	
spin	___
space	___
spy	___

[st]

# ___	
stove	___
stew	___
stop	___

[sk]

# ___	
sky	___
skip	___
ski	___

[sw]

# ___	
swamp	___
swim	___
sweet	___

[sn]

# ___	
snow	___
snake	___
snap	___

[sm]

# ___	
smell	___
smoke	___
small	___

[pl]

# ___	
play	___
plate	___
please	___

[fl]

# ___	
flag	___
fly	___
floor	___

continued

[bl]
#____
bloom ____
blind ____
blood ____

[gl]
#____
glue ____
glow ____
glass ____

[br]
#____
brain ____
brɔɔn ____
break ____

[fr]
#____
fruit ____
free ____
frog ____

[skw]
#____
squeak ____
square ____
squad ____

4;0

[z]
____ #
keys ____
please ____
buzz ____

[pr]
#____
pray ____
print ____
prune ____

[kr]
#____
crib ____
crow ____
cry ____

[dr]
#____
dry ____
drum ____
drop ____

[kl]
#____
clock ____
cloud ____
clue ____

178

4;6

[θ]
\# _____
think _____
thief _____
thick _____

[ð]
\# _____
that _____
this _____
them _____

[gr]
\# _____
grin _____
grass _____
grow _____

[sl]
\# _____
slam _____
sleep _____
slow _____

5;0

[tr]
\# _____
trout _____
truck _____
tree _____

[θr]
\# _____
three _____
throw _____
thread _____

[spr]
\# _____
spray _____
spread _____
spring _____

[str]
\# _____
street _____
straw _____
stream _____

[skr]
\# _____
screw _____
scratch _____
screen _____

[spl]
\# _____
splash _____
split _____
splurge _____

APPENDIX 3P
Calculation of Adjusted Age (AA)

A. Instructions

Use the formula below to calculate adjusted age for clients 24 months or younger who were born prematurely.

1. Adjusted Age Formula

Chronological age − Prematurity in weeks = Adjusted age

2. Example

5 months − 3 weeks premature = 4 months, 1 week old

APPENDIX 3Q
CALCULATION OF DEVELOPMENTAL AGE (DA)

A. Instructions

Use the formula below to calculate developmental age for clients with possible cognitive or intellectual limitations.

1. Verbal IQ or Standard Score

a. Client's verbal intelligence _____

b. Standard score (PPVT-R) _____

2. Developmental Age Formula

$$\frac{\text{Client's IQ or PPVT-R Standard Score} \times \text{CA in months}}{100} = \text{Developmental Age Level}$$

3. Example

$$\frac{82 \times 36}{100} = 29.52 \text{ months (30 months)}$$

APPENDIX 3R
Black English Vernacular (BEV)[1]

A. Instructions

Transcribe the client's speech. Place a check mark next to the client's BEV patterns on the assessment form that follows. BEV patterns are excluded from analysis of articulation and phonological disorders.

B. Assessment Scale for Black English Venacular (BEV)

Patterns	Examples
☐ Stopping	
[θ] → [t]	"thought" is "tought"
[ð] → [d]	"this" is "dis"
☐ Place changes between vowels and word finally	
[θ] → [f]	"bath" is "baf"
[ŋ] → [n]	"owing" is "owin"
[ð] → [v]	"bathing" is "baving"
☐ Devoicing at ends of words	
[b] → [p]	"slab" is "slap"
[d] → [t]	"bed" is "bet"
[g] → [k]	"bug" is "buk"
☐ Lowering of [ɪ] before nasals	
[ɪ] → [ɛ]	"pin" is "pen"
☐ Deletion	
V + [r] → V + ø	"more" is "mo"
CC# → Cø#	"nest" is "nes"
☐ Vowel nasalization and nasal deletion	
V + N → nasalized vowel	"tame" is "tã"

---

[1] The data source for this appendix is Cole and Taylor (1990).

APPENDIX 3S
Hawaiian Island Creole (HC)

A. Instructions

Transcribe the client's speech. Place a check mark next to the client's Hawaiian Island Creole patterns on the assessment form that follows. Exclude Hawaiian Island Creole patterns from analysis of articulation and phonological disorders.

B. Assessment Scale for Hawaiian Island Creole

Patterns	Examples
☐ Stopping	
[θ] → [t]	"thick" is "tick"
[ð] → [d]	"this" is "dis"
☐ Backing in environment of [r]	
[θr] → [tʃr]	"three" is "chree"
[tr] → [tʃr]	"tree" is "chree"
[str] → [ʃtrʒ]	"street" is "shtreet"
☐ Deletion	
V + [r] → V + schwa	"here" is "hea"
CC# → Cø#	"nest" is "nes"

---

[1] The data source for this appendix is Lyons (1994).

CHAPTER

4

Treatment Principles

The following topics are discussed in this chapter:

I. OVERVIEW OF TREATMENT

Four treatment principles are discussed in this chapter: purposes of treatment, goals (long- and short-term), treatment targets, and administrative decisions. In each section an introductory discussion is followed by a discussion of clients at specific stages in articulation and phonological development. The chapter concludes with brief summaries of complete treatment programs and a discussion of methods to evaluate treatment effectiveness.

II. PURPOSES OF TREATMENT

As discussed in Chapter 1, the client's stage of articulation and phonological development is more important than his or her chronological age when making decisions about clinical care. For convenience, the ways in which the general purpose of treatment changes depending on the client's stage of articulation and phonological development are presented in Table 4-1.

Early Intervention

Younger clients almost always receive articulation and phonological treatment within the framework of an early intervention program with a strong emphasis on language development (Bleile & Miller, in press). Several studies have demonstrated the effectiveness of early intervention on later developmental skills (Infant Health and Development Program, 1990; Bricker, Bailey, & Bruder, 1984; Ramey & Campbell, 1984; White, Mastrapierl, & Casto, 1984; Mantovani & Powers, 1991). The Infant Health and Development Program (1990), for example, after studying preterm at-risk infants at eight different clinical settings, found that the children who received early intervention had intelligence quotients (IQs) from 6.6 to 13.2 points higher than preterm children who received only routine follow-up care. The smaller gains in intelligence were obtained by children with the lowest birthweights, perhaps reflecting reduced potential for learning. A striking finding of the study was that preterm children who did not receive early intervention were 2.7 times more likely to have IQ scores in the mentally retarded range at 3 years of age than preterm children who did receive early intervention.

III. LONG-TERM GOALS

Long-term goals are the articulation and phonological behaviors that the client is expected to exhibit either at the end of treatment or after a designated time period, for example, a semester or school year.

A. Stage 1

The most common long-term treatment goal is for the client's articulation and phonological development to be appropriate for his or her chronological or developmental age. Adjusted ages should be used instead of chronological age for clients 2 years old

Table 4–1. Primary purposes of care at four different stages in articulation and phonological development.

Stages	Age Range in Typically Developing Children	Primary Purpose of Care
Stage 1	0–12 ms	Facilitate practice of vocal skills that serve as the basis for later speech development
Stage 2	12–24 ms	Facilitate the acquisition of sounds and syllables in specific words
Stage 3	2–5 yrs	Facilitate the elimination of errors affecting classes of sounds
Stage 4	>5 yrs	Facilitate the elimination of errors affecting late-acquired consonants, consonant clusters, and unstressed syllables in more difficult multisyllabic words

or younger who were born prematurely (see Chapter 3). Success or failure in achieving long-term goals typically is measured using age norms, although clinical judgment scales of severity represent a second possibility (see Chapter 3).

B. Stage 2

The most common long-term treatment goal is for the client's articulation and phonological development to be appropriate for his or her chronological or developmental age. Adjusted age should be used instead of chronological age for clients 2 years or younger who were born prematurely (see Chapter 3). Success or failure in achieving long-term goals is measured using age norms and/or judgments of severity of involvement (see Chapter 3).

C. Stage 3

The long-term treatment goal is for articulation and phonological development to be appropriate for the client's chronological or developmental age. Success or failure in achieving long-term goals is measured using age norms and measures of either severity of involvement or intelligibility (see Chapter 3).

D. Stage 4

The most common long-term treatment goal is for the client's articulation and phonological development to be appropriate for his or her chronological or developmental age (see Chapter 3). Success or failure in achieving long-term goals may be measured using any of the measures discussed in Chapter 3, including age norms, severity of involvement, and/or degree of intelligibility. Another possible long-term goal is to eliminate articulation and phonological errors that affect a client's happiness or social and educational development. This long-term goal would be appropriate, for example, for a client who was teased because of a [w] for [r] substitution or who experienced embarrassment when speaking to groups because of a frontal lisp. The success or failure in achieving this long-term goal might be determined at the client and/or family interview at the conclusion of treatment.

Family Education

Education about articulation and phonological disorders should be a long-term goal for all appropriate clients and their families. Major topics of discussion with families include the nature of the client's disorder, the client's current degree of disability, and the prognosis for future articulation and phonological development.

IV. SHORT-TERM GOALS

Short-term goals are the steps, each typically lasting from a few weeks to several months, through which long-term goals are achieved. The major short-term goals for clients at the four stages in articulation and phonological development are listed in Table 4-2.

A. Stage 1

There are two short-term goals for clients in Stage 1: increase opportunities to vocalize and facilitate the acquisition of developmentally advanced vocalizations.

Table 4-2. Short-term goals for clients at four different stages in articulation and phonological development.

Stages	Short-term Goal
Stage 1	Increase opportunities to vocalize
	Facilitate acquisition of developmentally advanced vocalizations
Stages 2 and 3	Reduction in homonyms
	Reduction of variability
	Maximization of established speech ability
	Elimination of errors affecting sound classes
Stage 4	Facilitation of late-acquired consonants, consonant clusters, and unstressed syllables in more difficult multisyllabic words

1. **Increase Opportunities to Vocalize.** This short-term goal seeks to increase the client's opportunities to vocalize. It is an appropriate short-term goal for hospitalized clients and those who are victims of environmental neglect or abuse. Increasing vocalizations can be pursued as early as the first few months of life, as a client awakens more frequently and becomes more alert. A possible short-term goal, for example, might be to provide opportunities for a hospitalized client to vocalize on waking or before napping, and/or to train a parent how to interact better with his or her child. In most settings, vocal stimulation is carried out by a family member, although in a hospital setting this task might be undertaken by a speech-language clinician, an aide, or a nurse.

2. **Acquisition of Developmentally Advanced Vocalizations.** This short-term goal seeks to facilitate the acquisition of developmentally advanced vocalizations. It is an appropriate short-term goal for clients who either are at risk for or have already experienced delays in articulation and phonological development. As above, facilitating the acquisition of vocalizations can be pursued as early as the first months of life, as the client awakens more frequently. A short-term goal, for example, might be to facilitate nonreduplicated babbling for a client whose developmentally most advanced vocalization is reduplicated babbling.

B. Stages 2 and 3

There are four possible short-term goals for clients in Stages 2 or 3: reduce homonyms, reduce variability, maximize established speech abilities, and eliminate errors affecting classes of sounds.

When the Goal Is Nothing New

There are at least three situations in which the short-term goal of treatment is to extend the client's use of existing articulation and phonological abilities rather than to facilitate the acquisition of new sounds and syllables. The first situation is when the clinician affords opportunities to vocalize to a client in Stage 1 who may have experienced either deprivation through neglect or as a result of lengthy hospitaliza-

---

tions. The second situation is when the expressive vocabulary of a client in Stage 2 or 3 contains many homonyms and the clinician "floods" the vocabulary with words that result in increased numbers of homonyms. The third situation is when the clinician helps construct a larger expressive vocabulary for a client in Stage 2 or 3 using existing articulation and phonological skills.

1. **Reduce Homonyms.** This short-term goal seeks to reduce the percentage of homonyms (words that sound alike, but have different meanings) in the client's speech. The presence of homonyms is normal in both children's and adults' speech, but unusual numbers of homonyms in small expressive vocabularies may severely interfere with communication. A client with a 10-word expressive vocabulary, for example, 7 of which are pronounced as [bi], is likely to experience difficulty conveying his or her wants and needs, especially when speaking to unfamiliar adults. There are two general approaches to reducing homonyms: eliminate errors causing homonyms and "flooding."

   a. **Eliminate Errors Causing Homonyms.** This approach seeks to eliminate error patterns or sound class errors causing homonyms (Ingram, 1989). A client, for example, who pronounced "cookie," "Tom," "kite," and "toe" as [di] might have reduction of Fronting as a short-term goal, so that "cookie" and "kite" would then be pronounced with an initial [k] and "Tom" and "toe" would be pronounced with an initial [t].

   b. **Flooding.** This approach seeks to reduce the number of homonyms by causing the client to reorganize his or her articulation and phonological systems (Bleile & Miller, 1994). Somewhat ironically, flooding works by facilitating the acquisition of words which results in an increased number of homonyms in the client's speech. The increase in the number of homonyms results in communicative breakdown and frustration, inducing speech changes as the client is forced to attempt new pronunciations in order to communicate.

Flooding is an experimental procedure that I have used successfully as a last resort with clients whose speech contained many homonyms and who did not improve by other means. Before attempting flooding, I would first attempt eliminating errors affecting error patterns, perhaps using request for clarification activities described in Chapter 5. If this was not successful, I would attempt flooding. A client whose expressive vocabulary was dominated by words pronounced as [di], for example, would be taught words that the assessment indicated would also be pronounced as [di]. The clinician would then engage the client in the type of request for clarification activities described in Chapter 5. To illustrate, the client might say [di] as a request for a cookie, and the clinician might give him or her a spoon, key, plate, or other object that the client also pronounces as [di].

Veto Power

Treatment with clients in Stage 2 is based on a lexical approach that is designed primarily to facilitate the acquisition of sounds and syllables in specific words. If a treatment goal is to help a client acquire [p], for example, he or she would be exposed to many different objects and names of favorite persons that begin with [p]. Next, the clinician and the client's caregivers select two to three objects and names in which the client shows the greatest interest. These words receive additional attention during treatment, and the caregivers attempt to use the words at home. The client, of course, has veto power over any words selected in a lexical approach. An adult, for example, may select [p] in "pie" for treatment, but the client instead may elect to say only [p] in "papa." In this situation, the clinician follows the client's lead and shifts the focus of treatment to [p] in "papa." It is important for the client's caregivers to be aware of such word changes to provide the client as consistent a learning environment as possible.

2. **Reduce Variability.** This short-term goal seeks to reduce the client's alternate pronunciations of words and sounds. Reduction in variability is appropriate for clients in Stage 2 and some less advanced clients in Stage 3 who appear extremely variable in their pronunciation of a sound or sounds. Variability is a hallmark of many clients with articulation and phonological disorders, especially clients with Down syndrome.

There are two types of variability: intraword variability and interword variability. **Intraword variability** is variation in the pronunciation of a sound or sounds in the same word. A client whose speech showed intraword variability, for example, might say the initial sound in "bee" as [b], [p], or [mb]. **Interword variability** is variation in the pronunciation of a sound or sounds in different words. A client whose speech showed interword variability, for example, might say [b] as [b] in "bee," as [d] in "bay," and as [p] in "boo." Both intra- and interword variability interfere with communication. More positively, however, variability suggests that better pronunciation of a sound is within the client's phonetic abilities, even though the client may not yet be able to produce it correctly on all occasions. When the short-term goal is to reduce variability, the general clinical strategy is to use facilitative techniques that encourage the client to produce the most developmentally advanced variant of the sound.

3. **Maximize Established Speech Abilities.** This short-term goal seeks to maximize the client's existing articulation and phonological abilities (Bleile & Miller, 1994). Maximizing established speech abilities is appropriate for clients in Stage 2 for whom the major treatment goal is vocabulary building and for less advanced clients in Stage 3 who are temporarily "stalled" in either articulation or phonological development. This short-term goal involves increasing the use of the client's existing abilities to pronounce sounds, syllables, and word shapes. Use of established speech abilities reduces the speech complexity of learning new words, particularly if the client's speech is organized around word recipes or selectively (see Chapter 3). The constructed words should be pragmatically useful and contain well-established sounds, syllables, and word shapes. If the client's established phonetic inventory, for example, contained the CV syllable [ki], the

clinician would discuss with the client's parents whether the word "key" has functional value for the client. If so, "key" would receive special emphasis during treatment while the client's family attempted to facilitate use of the word at home.

Why Distinctive Features and Error Patterns?

Distinctive feature and error pattern approaches were developed to speed remediation through generalization of treatment results from a treated sound to untreated sounds. A distinctive feature approach organizes sounds into classes based on shared acoustic and articulatory features; the hoped-for result of treatment is that generalization will occur from the treated sounds to other sounds that share similar features. Facilitating acquisition of [f], for example, may facilitate the client's acquisition of other fricatives. An error pattern approach organizes sounds according to the errors they typically undergo; the hoped-for result of treating one sound is that the results will generalize to other sounds that undergo the same error. Which approach facilitates better generalization — use of distinctive features or error patterns? I do not believe there is yet sufficient research to answer that important question.

---

4. **Eliminate Errors Affecting Sound Classes.** This short-term goal seeks to eliminate errors that affect entire classes of sounds. Elimination of errors affecting sound classes is appropriate for all clients in Stages 2 and 3 whose speech contains articulation and phonological errors affecting sound classes. Two closely related approaches are used to eliminate errors affecting sound classes: distinctive feature approaches and error pattern approaches.

a. **Distinctive Feature Approaches.** In a distinctive feature approach, sounds are remediated based on their membership in a sound class. The sound classes most often used for this purpose are the various place, manner, and voicing categories found in a consonant chart.

Some clinicians remediate all sounds in a sound class (Blodgett & Miller, 1989). For example, a clinician might treat all velar consonants in the speech of a client who pronounced velar consonants as alveolar consonants. Other clinicians recommend treating fewer sounds within sound classes (Elbert, Powell, & Schwartz, 1991; Williams, 1991). I remediate from two sounds up to 50% of the sounds in a sound class in the hope that the treatment results will generalize to other sounds sharing the distinctive feature. For example, treatment for a client who pronounced [k] and [g] as alveolar consonants in the beginning of syllables might focus on facilitating acquisition of [k] in the hope that the client will generalize the ability to produce stop consonants in the velar region to other velar consonants. The motivation to remediate only a few sounds in a sound class is that it saves time for the clients who generalize and costs no additional time for those who do not. Word probes such as those described in Appendix 2A might be used to determine whether generalization has occurred.

b. **Error Pattern Approaches.** An error pattern approach seeks to eliminate sounds based on their membership in error patterns. As with the distinctive feature approach, some clinicians provide treatment to all sounds affected by an error pattern, whereas others, the author included, remediate from two sounds up to 50% of the sounds affected by an error pattern in the hope that the treatment results will generalize to other sounds affected by the error pattern. A client, for example, might have a Fronting error pattern in the beginning of syllables, and treatment might focus on remediating [k] in that syllable position in the hope that the results will generalize to [g] and [ŋ].

An important issue to consider is which error patterns should be selected for remediation. I typically select error patterns for remediation that are either frequent (50–75% of all possible occurrences) or present (25–49% of all occurrences). (See Table 3–2 for categories based on whole numbers rather than percentages.) I tend to avoid error patterns that are highly frequent (75–100% of all possible occurrences), because their remediation often is too time-consuming for younger clients. I also tend to avoid remediating error patterns that are disappearing (1–24%), because in most situations the client appears to be overcoming them without treatment.

C. Stage 4

The major short-term goal for clients in Stage 4 is to facilitate the elimination of errors affecting late-acquired consonants, consonant clusters, and unstressed syllables in more difficult multisyllabic words. A client, for example, might be limited to word-initial syllables beginning with a consonant (C) followed by a vowel (V). A possible goal for this client would be to facilitate the acquisition of syllables that begin with consonant clusters (Bernhardt, in press; Bernhardt & Gilbert, 1992). Most often, emerging (10–49% correct) consonants, consonant clusters, and unstressed syllables are selected as short-term goals (see Table 3–3 for categories based on whole numbers rather than percentages). Rare (1–9% correct) and absent (0% correct) consonants, consonant clusters, and unstressed syllables often prove extrememly challenging for most clients. Short-term goals are seldom mastered (90–100% correct), acquired (75–89% correct), or present (50–74%) for late-acquired consonants, consonant clusters, and unstressed syllables because the client appears well on the way to having acquired these sounds and syllables without treatment.

V. OVERVIEW OF TREATMENT TARGETS

Although long- and short-term goals give direction to clinical endeavors, treatment targets are the actual sounds and syllables through which change in a client's articulation and phonological systems is facilitated. For example, a long-term goal might be, "Articulation and phonological development will be appropriate for the client's age," and the short-term goal might be, "Elimination of Fronting in the beginning of syllables." The treatment target is the sound (or sounds) through which the restriction on velar consonants (Fronting) in syllable-initial position is eliminated. To illustrate, the clinician might choose [k] as the treatment target, hoping that the results of treating

[k] will generalize to other velar consonants. The major issues that arise in considering treatment targets include selecting treatment targets, determining how many treatment targets should be treated, changing treatment targets, and choosing linguistic levels and phonetic environments.

Clinical Philosophy

Treatment targets are selected based on the clinician's treatment philosophy in conjunction with the clinician's perception of the nature of the client's articulation and phonological disorder. For example, a clinician who believes that intelligibility is of primary importance is likely to select treatment targets that have the greatest impact on that aspect of articulation and phonological development. (See Chapter 3 for the effects of consonants and error patterns on perceived intelligibility.) Similarly, a clinician who believes that degree of developmental delay is of primary importance is likely to select treatment targets that have the greatest impact on the client's development delay (see Chapter 3 for age norms). Finally, a clinician who believes that the social and educational impact of articulation and phonological disorders is of primary importance is likely to select treatment targets that have the greatest effect on the client's social and educational well-being.

VI. SELECTING TREATMENT TARGETS

Most often, the clinician selects treatment targets that the client demonstrates some capacity to produce. Four possible methods to determine whether a client is able to produce a treatment target are listed in Table 4–3 and described below.

A. Stimulability

Stimulability is the client's ability to imitate a treatment target (see Section V in Chapter 3 for assessment procedures). Stimulability indicates that the client is physically able to produce the sound. Treatment seeks to generalize use of the sound from imitation to spontaneous speech.

Table 4–3. Four methods to select treatment targets.

Criteria	Definitions
Stimulability	The client is stimulable for the treatment target
Emerging sound	The client can produce the treatment target in either several phonetic environments or one key phonetic environment
Key word	The client can produce the treatment target in one or a few selected words
Phonetic placement and shaping	The client can produce the treatment target through phonetic placement or through shaping an existing sound

B. Emerging Sound

An emerging sound is one that is produced correctly on 10 to 49% of all occasions in one or more phonetic environments (the phonetic environment is called a key environment if the client is only able to produce the treatment target in a single phonetic environment). An example of an emerging sound is [k] in the speech of a client who correctly produced [k] in word-initial position in 2 of 10 words (20%). If the client is able to produce a treatment target in several phonetic environments, treatment seeks to increase the frequency with which the sound is produced. If the client is only able to produce the sound in one key environment, treatment seeks to generalize success from that phonetic environment to other phonetic environments.

Selecting Treatment Targets

Whenever possible, most clinicians select treatment targets that are stimulable, that the client produces in one or more words or phonetic environments, or that the client produces with the help of phonetic placement and shaping techniques. Because the client already has some capacity to produce the treatment target, the clinician can more quickly shift treatment to generalization of the treatment target to other

---

words or phonetic environments, rather than focusing treatment on the often frustrating and time-consuming task of teaching the client to pronounce a treatment target that the client shows no capacity to produce in any circumstance.

C. Key Word

A key word is a word in which the client successfully produces the treatment target. Although any word can be a key word, many times key words have special significance for a client, such as being the name of a favorite toy or person. Treatment based on a key word seeks to generalize success in producing the sound to other words (see Section XII for discussion of the Paired-stimuli [key word] treatment program).

D. Phonetic Placement and Shaping

Phonetic placement involves the physical placement of a client's articulators into position to produce a sound. Phonetic placement of [t], for example, entails detailed instructions that guide the client to quickly touch the alveolar ridge with the tongue tip. Shaping involves developing a new sound from a sound already in the client's phonetic inventory. Shaping techniques, for example, provide a series of steps through which a [t] might be shaped into [s]. Treatment seeks to generalize success in performing phonetic placement and shaping techniques to spontaneous speech. Phonetic placement and shaping techniques are provided in Appendix 5C.

E. Stage 1

The most appropriate treatment targets for clients in Stage 1 are those that are emerging and for which the client is stimulable.

F. Stages 2 and 3

The most appropriate treatment targets for clients in Stages 2 and 3 are those that are stimulable and emerging. The next most-preferred treatment targets are those that are either emerging, stimulable, or in key words or key environments. Treatment targets may also be rarely produced sounds, although the likelihood exists that the client will find such targets more frustrating. For this reason, the preferred clinical strategy is to monitor rarely occurring sounds and treat them after they are produced correctly more frequently.

G. Stage 4

As with clients in earlier stages of articulation and phonological development, the most appropriate treatment targets for clients in Stage 4 are treatment targets that are stimulable, emerging, or in key words. Differing from clients in earlier stages, the clinician can also target more rarely produced sounds, because many clients in Stage 4 are able to tolerate less immediate treatment success. The often greater cognitive maturation of clients in Stage 4 also allows the clinician to utilize shaping and phonetic placement techniques. Even so, such techniques are likely to require more patience and attention than is possible for clients in Stage 4 who are immature or who experience behavioral problems, intellectual deficits, or cognitive impairments.

VII. MOST AND LEAST KNOWLEDGE METHODS

Most often, treatment targets require the client to acquire new sounds and syllables. Two methods can be used to determine how similar treatment targets should be compared to the client's current articulation and phonological abilities: the most knowledge method and the least knowledge method.

A. Most Knowledge Method

The most knowledge method is a traditional criterion used to choose treatment targets. In this method, treatment targets differ minimally from the sounds the client already produces (Elbert & Gierut, 1986). This means that the client has a great deal of knowledge about the treatment target, because he or she already is producing many features of the treatment target in other sounds. For example, within the most knowledge method the treatment target for a client whose phonetic inventory contained one oral stop ([p]) and no fricatives would likely be another oral stop — perhaps a sound that differed only in voicing (e.g., [b]) or in place of production (e.g., [t] or [k]). The close similarity between the client's existing abilities and the treatment target is intended to ensure that the new sound will be acquired without great frustration for the client (Van Riper, 1978). A possible limitation of a most knowledge method is that treatment must proceed in small increments, which proves time-consuming with clients who have multiple articulation and phonological errors. To acquire the entire set of oral stops, for example, the above client's treatment targets would include [b], [t], [d], [k], and [g].

Least Knowledge: Distinctive Features or Error Patterns?

The least knowledge method is closely associated with the use of a distinctive feature approach, but it might also be undertaken within an error pattern framework. For example, a client's speech might contain the following characteristics: stopping, a well-established [b], no alveolar consonants, and stimulability for [f] and [s]. In a more traditional most knowledge method, the likely treatment target in this situation is [f], because that sound is most similar to [b] (a labial consonant). In a least knowledge method, the likely treatment target is [s], because [s] facilitates the acquisition of a new place of production.

B. Least Knowledge Method

In a least knowledge method, treatment targets differ from the client's existing abilities by multiple features (Elbert & Gierut, 1986; Powell, 1991). The client described above whose speech contained one oral stop ([p]) and no fricatives, for example, might have [z] as a treatment target. The essential idea underlying a least knowledge method is that treatment targets should afford the client the opportunity to acquire skills needed to produce more than single sounds. In acquiring [z], for example, the client also acquires a new contrast in place of production (bilabial and alveolar), a new voicing contrast (voiceless and voiced), and a new manner of production (stop and fricative). Presently, the least knowledge method is a relatively new proposal, and its effectiveness has been studied only with a small number of subjects. The results of these investigations, however, appear promising for the least knowledge method as an alternative to the more traditional most knowledge method for clients whose speech contain multiple errors.

C. Stage 1

Although in principle a least knowledge method is possible for clients in Stage 1, all the clients I have treated have only responded to a more traditional most knowledge method.

D. Stages 2 and 3

A least knowledge method is often appropriate for clients in Stages 2 and 3 because generalization to untreated sounds and syllables may occur more quickly than with a most knowledge method. The following procedure is helpful in deciding whether to use a most or least knowledge method:

Select treatment targets based on the criteria listed in Section VI (key word, stimulable, or emerging in at least one key phonetic environment).

If more than one treatment target meets the above criteria, select the sound that is least similar to the sounds the client is currently able to produce (least knowledge method).

If the client fails to make progress using a least knowledge method, select treatment targets more similar to the sounds the client is currently able to produce (most knowledge method).

E. Stage 4

A least knowledge approach becomes less clinically relevant for clients in Stage 4, because generalization to untreated sounds is less relevant when errors arise only in a few late-acquired consonants, consonant clusters, and unstressed syllables in more difficult multisyllabic words.

VIII. NUMBER OF TREATMENT TARGETS

Typically, only one treatment target is facilitated per session. This is because many clients find it confusing to receive treatment on more than one treatment target in a single session. The exceptions to this general rule are clients who require a flexible approach (see next section) or when a clinician chooses a multiple phoneme approach (see discussion of articulation programs later in this chapter).

More than one treatment target can be facilitated over the same period of weeks or months. Two general strategies are used to help decide how many treatment targets to facilitate simultaneously: training deep and training wide (Elbert & Gierut, 1986). **Training deep** provides intensive treatment on one or two treatment targets, which allows proportionally more attention to be devoted to each treatment target than is the case when a greater number of treatment targets are selected. **Training wide** provides treatment on three or more treatment targets, which offers the client more opportunities to discover relationships between targets than if a training deep strategy is selected. A client who receives treatment on [p], [d], and [s], for example, is being exposed to contrasts in place of production (bilabial and alveolar), voicing (voiced and voiceless), and manner (stop and fricative).

A. Stages 1 Through 3

Training wide is appropriate with clients in the first three stages of articulation and phonological development due to these clients' greater number of errors and shorter attention spans.

B. Stage 4

Although training wide is appropriate for all clients, a training deep approach often appears better suited to clients in Stage 4 who have sufficient attention spans to concentrate on a treatment target for an extended time period.

IX. CHANGING TREATMENT TARGETS

An important consideration is determining when to change from one treatment target to another during the course of treatment. In this book, three criteria for changing treatment targets are flexibility, time, and percentage.

A. Flexibility

If a flexible criterion is used, a treatment target is facilitated until the client becomes disinterested, at which point another treatment target is facilitated. An illustration of a flexible criterion is the statement: "Treatment for [b] will continue for as long as the client's interest is sustained."

B. Time

If a time criterion is used, a certain amount of treatment time (typically, 60 minutes) is devoted to each target (Hodson, 1989). After that time is completed, treatment shifts to another treatment target. After treatment for all targets is completed (called a cycle), the treatment targets are treated again (a second cycle). Cycles are repeated until all treatment targets are remediated, which typically requires from three to four cycles (approximately 1 year of treatment). An illustration of a time criterion is the statement, "Treatment for [t] will be provided for 1 hour in cycle 1."

C. Percentage

If a percentage criterion is used, a treatment target is facilitated until a certain percentage of correct production is reached. An illustration of a percentage criterion is the statement: "Correct production of [s] in word initial position 75% of the time."

Linguistic Generalization

Some clients easily generalize the results of treatment to untreated sounds, linguistic levels, and words. For most clients, however, generalization happens more slowly and less completely. Although no procedures are "guaranteed" to promote generalization in all clients, distinctive feature approaches, error pattern approaches, least knowledge methods, and training wide maximize the chance that generalization will occur to other sounds. When the short-term goal is reduction of Fronting, for example, the hope is that the results of success on one sound will generalize to other sounds affected by the Fronting pattern. If, however, generalization does not occur, the clinician needs to treat the individual sounds affected by the Fronting pattern.

D. Stage 1

I have found a flexible approach extremely useful with clients in Stage 1 and other clients whose cognitive abilities do not permit successful performance using more structured criteria. For example, the short-term goal might be to facilitate reduplicated babbling, and the possible treatment targets might be reduplicated CV syllables that begin with [b], [d], or [m]. The clinician would then come to each treatment session ready to facilitate any of the treatment targets, depending on the client's inclinations.

E. Stage 2

A time approach is an appropriate criterion for many clients in Stage 2. For example, a clinician might provide 1 hour of treatment for each treatment target. Clients who lack the cognitive and attention abilities for a time criterion are treated using a flexible approach. For example, the client's short-term goal might be to eliminate Prevocalic Voicing, and the possible treatment targets might be [t] in "tea" and "toe," [p] in "pie," and [f] in "food." The clinician would then come to each treatment session ready to facilitate any of the treatment targets.

F. Stage 3

Time is an appropriate criterion for changing treatment targets with the vast majority of clients in Stage 3. For example, the speech of a client in transition between Stages 3 and 4 might contain Gliding and errors affecting several individual sounds, including Stopping of [s] and Devoicing of word-final [b]. A cycle for such a client might include an hour each of treatment for [l], [r], [s], and word-final [b]. Lastly, clients in Stage 3 who lack the cognitive and attention abilities needed for a time criterion are provided treatment using the flexible approach described for clients in Stages 1 and 2. Clients in Stage 3 with exceptionally good attention skills are provided treatment using a percentage criterion.

G. Stage 4

A percentage criterion is appropriate for most clients in Stage 4, although a time criterion may be needed for clients in Stage 4 who have limited attention and cognitive abilities. For example, a cycle for a client in Stage 4 might include an hour each of treatment for [s], [r], and unstressed syllables in multisyllabic words.

> ### Generalization to Other Settings and Persons
>
> Generalization to other persons and settings is facilitated through treatment activities that reflect real-life situations and use real words of high functional value to the client. The following ideas help to promote generalization to other settings and persons:
>
> - Hold frequent meetings with caregivers and other professionals to keep them informed about treatment goals and progress.
>
> - Have the client's caregivers occasionally attend and assist in treatment sessions.
>
> - With clients in Stages 3 and 4, give the caregiver a list of 10 words containing a target sound and ask him or her to spend 2 minutes a day having the client say each word (to avoid the caregiver becoming "a teacher," do not provide this suggestion until the client is approximately 80% correct in the clinic setting in producing the treatment target at the word level).
>
> - With clients in Stages 3 and 4, prepare a 2-minute audio tape of words containing the client's treatment targets and ask the client's parent to play it to the client.
>
> - With clients in Stages 3 and 4, ask the caregiver to place stickers around the house as reminders of treatment targets.

X. LINGUISTIC LEVEL AND PHONETIC ENVIRONMENTS

Treatment targets typically are introduced in a single linguistic level in either one or two phonetic environments. The possible linguistic levels are isolated sounds, nonsense syllables, words, phrases, sentences, and spontaneous speech; the possible phonetic environments are word positions (initial, medial, final) and syllable positions (syllable initial, final, intervocalic, stressed and unstressed syllable, etc.).

A. Stage 1

Information in this section is not appropriate for clients in Stage 1.

B. Stages 2 Through 4

1. **Linguistic Level.** The preferred level for introducing treatment targets for clients in Stages 2 through 4 is the isolated word, because it is the lowest linguistic level that most closely approximates the skills the client uses outside the clinic setting. The exception to this general rule occurs when phonetic placement and shaping techniques are employed to introduce a treatment target to a client in Stage 4. More often, however, isolated sounds and nonsense syllables serve best as prompts during treatment for selected clients in Stage 3 and with most clients in Stage 4 who experience failure at the word level. If the client, for example, experiences failure with [d] in "dog," the clinician might prompt, "This is the [di] sound. Say [di]. Good. Now say [dog]."

   If a client already successfully produces a treatment target at the word level, treatment targets can be introduced at the level of the phrase, sentence, or spontaneous speech. A client, for example, might be asked to tell a story based on characters whose names contain the treatment target. Alternately, a client and clinician might play a barrier game in which the objects contain the treatment target (see Chapter 5 for additional suggestions for activities to facilitate treatment targets in phrases, sentences, and spontaneous speech).

   ### Changing Linguistic Levels

   Generally, treatment continues at one linguistic level until the client is able to produce the treatment target correctly 75% of the time before beginning treatment on the next higher linguistic level. A client, for example, should produce word-initial [t] correctly 75% of the time at the level of the isolated word before beginning treat-
   continued

> ment for the sound at the phrase level. The criterion of 75% is chosen because at that point the sound is acquired and, in most cases, is likely to progress to 100% correct without additional treatment. When the client is able to produce all of his or her treatment targets correctly 75 to 90% of the time in spontaneous speech, treatment is generally discontinued; the higher percentage is used if the clinician is concerned that the client will "regress" after treatment is ended, as happens too frequently over the long months of summer vacation (Kumai, 1994, personal communication).

2. **Phonetic Environments.** Phonetic environment (syllable position, word position, and nearby sounds) is critically important to the production of many sounds. The most likely phonetic environments in which to introduce treatment targets are listed in Table 4–4 (Bleile, 1991b). However, as with

Table 4–4. "Best bets" for environments within which to establish treatment targets.

Treatment Targets	Environments
All treatment targets	Establish in CV, CVCV, or VC syllables
All treatment targets	Establish in stressed syllables
Consonants	Except for the instances noted below, establish consonants in the beginning of words
Voiced	Establish either between vowels or in the beginning of words and syllables
Voiceless	Establish at the end of syllables and words
Velar stops	Establish at the end of words or at the beginning of words before a back vowel
Alveolar stops	Establish at the beginning of words before front vowels
Voiced fricatives	Establish between vowels

Source: From *Child Phonology: A Book of Exercises for Students* (p. 78) by K. Bleile, (1991b), San Diego, CA: Singular Publishing Group, with permission.

most clinical enterprises, the clinician does best to follow the client's lead in selecting both the number and types of phonetic environments in which to introduce treatment targets. If, for example, the client is more successful producing velar stops between vowels, then treatment should begin by facilitating velar stops in that position. Similarly, if the client appears stimulable for [t] in both word-initial and word-final positions, the clinician may consider beginning treatment in both positions.

XI. ADMINISTRATIVE DECISIONS

Treatment requires the clinician to make administrative decisions about the organization of treatment sessions, including whether to provide treatment individually or in groups, the frequency and length of sessions, types of activities, and length of individual treatment activities.

A. Types of Sessions

Treatment can be provided either in individual or group sessions. Individual sessions consist of a single client and are often preferred during the early stages of treatment when the clinician is introducing new treatment targets. Group sessions typically consist of three to five clients of similar ages and developmental levels and are often preferred in the middle and late stages of therapy, when goals shift from introducing new treatment targets to helping the client to generalize and maintain what has been learned.

B. Frequency of Sessions

Treatment for clients at all levels of articulation and phonological development typically is provided from two to five times a week. Some evidence exists that intensive therapy (four to five times a week) is slightly more efficient for clients in Stage 4 than less intensive therapy (twice a week) for a longer number of weeks (Bernthal & Bankson, 1993).

C. Length of Sessions

Individual therapy sessions range from 10 to 15 minutes to 1 hour. Group sessions typically range from 30 to 45 minutes.

D. Length of Activities in Sessions

Individual activities in sessions may last from less than a minute to nearly 30 minutes.

E. Format of Activities

There are four basic types of activities: drill, drill play, structured play, and play (Shriberg & Kwiatkowski, 1982).

1. **Drill.** Drill involves the clinician presenting material for mass practice by the client in activities such as repeating lists of words, naming pictures, and so on.

2. **Drill Play.** Drill play involves drills presented in the context of games such as spinning wheels, game boards, and so on.

3. **Structured Play.** Structured play is drill play presented in play-like activities such as playing house, shopping, parking toy cars in a garage, and so on.

4. **Play.** Play is child-oriented activities during which acquisition of targets is facilitated during the course of the activities.

Maintenance

Sometimes treatment success does not last after the client is discharged. With younger clients, the most important means of maintaining hard-won treatment successes after discharge is securing the cooperation of the client's family. This is accomplished through frequent meetings during which the purposes and goals of treatment are carefully explained and, if needed, home programs are developed. With clients in later stages of articulation and phonological development, both family involvement and ongoing exercises throughout treatment designed to develop the client's self-monitoring skills are the best guarantees that treatment gains will not be lost.

F. Stage 1

Decisions about treatment sessions are arrived at in conjunction with the client's caregivers. The options for treatment sessions and activities are to provide treatment on an individual or group basis from two to five times a week. Individual sessions typically last from 5 to 15 minutes, and group sessions typically last approximately 30 minutes. The client's attention for specific activities in treatment sessions typically ranges from a few seconds to 1 to 2 minutes. The preferred format for activities is play.

G. Stage 2

Decisions about treatment sessions are arrived at in conjunction with the client's caregivers. The options for treatment sessions and activities are to provide treatment individually or in early intervention groups from two to five times a week. Individual sessions typically last from 20 to 30 minutes, and early intervention sessions typically last approximately from 30 to 45 minutes. The client's attention for specific activities in treatment sessions typically ranges from a few minutes to 10 minutes. The preferred format for activities is play.

H. Stage 3

Decisions about treatment sessions are arrived at in conjunction with the client's caregivers. The options for treatment sessions and activities are to provide treatment in individual or group sessions from two to five times a week. Individual and group sessions typically last from 30 to 45 minutes. Individual activities in treatment sessions may last up to 10 minutes. The preferred formats for activities are structured play and drill play. Research indicates that drill play is more effective and efficient with clients in Stage 3 than structured play and is equally as effective as drill (Shriberg & Kwiatowski, 1982a).

I. Stage 4

The options for treatment sessions and activities are to provide treatment from two to five times a week in individual or group sessions. Individual sessions typically last from 30 to 45 minutes, and group sessions typically last approximately 45 minutes to 1 hour. Individual activities in treatment sessions are likely to last 10 to 15 minutes. The preferred formats for activities are drill play and, with more mature clients, drill.

XII. COMPLETE INTERVENTION PROGRAMS

A number of complete intervention programs have been developed to treat clients with articulation and phonological disorders. Although these programs are sometimes used in their entirety, more often clinicians borrow an idea here and adapt a procedure there as clinical need arises. The following is a summary of the major intervention programs presently in use in English-speaking countries. The programs are organized into two subsections: articulation (motor) and phonology (language) (Bernthal & Bankson, 1993). Before attempting any of the programs summarized below, the reader is referred to the references for detailed explanations of principles and procedures.

Articulation and Phonological Programs

Although there are crucial differences between articulation and phonological programs, few would debate that speech involves both motor control (articulation) and language knowledge (phonology). Instead, the debate in our field is over the relative importance of these two concepts in the remediation of speech disorders.

A. Articulation Programs

Articulation programs share the assumption that speech problems are largely motoric in origin — a reasonable assumption, considering that these programs were largely developed to treat school-age children with errors affecting individual, late-acquired consonants and consonant clusters. The most influential articulation programs are the Van Riper approach, the Paired-stimuli program, the Sensory-motor program, Multiple Phoneme program, and the Motoric Automatization of Articulatory Performance Program.

1. Van Riper Approach (Traditional Approach)

a. Reference

Van Riper, C. (1978). *Speech correction: Principles and methods* (6th ed.). Englewood Cliffs, NJ: Prentice-Hall.

b. Overview

The Van Riper approach (also called the Traditional Approach), first published in the mid-1930s, is a compilation of clinical ideas developed during the early years of the 20th century. The assumptions underlying the Van Riper approach are that articulation and phonological errors may result from both faulty perception abilities and inadequate oral motor skills. Treatment consists of both perceptual and production training. Production training often begins with isolated sounds or nonsense syllables in order to avoid interference with existing "speech habits." Treatment proceeds in small increments (a most knowledge method), so that the client may experience as much success as possible.

c. Comment

Throughout most of the 20th century the Van Riper approach was the most widely accepted clinical model for treating articulation and phonological disorders, but it declined in popularity as clinical populations grew ever younger and more severely involved. Still, the Van Riper approach remains a viable clinical alternative with many clients in Stage 4, the clinical population for which it was chiefly intended. The Van Riper approach is less successful with clients in Stages 2 and 3, both as a model of articulation and phonological disorders and as a set of practical treatment procedures.

2. Paired-stimuli (Key Word) Program

a. Reference

Irwin, J., & Weston, A. (1975). The paired-stimuli monograph. *Acta Symbolica, 6,* 1–76.

> ### Evolution of an Idea
>
> The founders of our profession knew that sounds belonged to sound classes, although they tended not to emphasize this in clinical practice because it was not pertinent to the care of their clients, the vast majority of whom experienced speech problems affecting individual consonants and consonant clusters. Interest in sound classes grew in the late 1960s and 1970s, as the caseloads of speech-language clinicans increasingly came to include preschoolers, the majority of whom had errors affecting entire sound classes. At that point, clinicians became concerned about the enormous amount of time required if each sound needed to be treated individually.

b. Overview

The Paired-stimuli program was developed based on principles of behavioral psychology. The assumption underlying the Paired-stimuli program is that success in producing a sound embedded in a word can be generalized to other words containing the sound. A key word contains a treatment target that is produced correctly 9 out of 10 times in either the initial or final position. If a key word is not found during the assessment, the clinician facilitates the acquisition of the treatment target and then transfers it to a key word. The clinician then selects 10 words that have the same error in the same word position. A picture of the key word is placed in the center of the table and the training words are placed around it. The client is instructed to say the key word, which is then reinforced, followed by a training word, which is not reinforced unless it is produced correctly. Training proceeds until all of the training words are produced (called one training string). Three training strings are completed in one half-hour training session.

c. Comment

The most interesting aspect of the Paired-stimuli program is that it provides a means to generalize correct production of a treatment target in one word to other words. Although conceived as a behaviorist program, the Paired-stimuli program might be modified by deemphasizing the reinforcement aspects of the program and offering the client instructions that rely more on his or her linguistic abilities. A session, for example, might begin with activities to facilitate the client's awareness of the treatment target and to help the client to identify the correct production of the treatment target in a key word, for example, [s] in "sun." Next, the clinician might place pictures of the key word and training words in a circle, as described above, explaining, "Let's play a game. In the game, first you say 'sun' and then one of the other words, going around the circle until we say all the words. Try to say the words on the outside with the same snake sound as 'sun.' " The instructions, of course, could be modified, simplified, or expanded based on the client's interests and level of cognitive development.

3. Sensory-motor Program

a. References

McDonald, E. (1964). *Articulation testing and treatment: A sensory-motor approach.* Pittsburgh: Stanwix House.

Shine, R. (1989). Articulatory production training: A sensory-motor approach. In. N. Creaghead, P. Newman, & W. Secord (Eds.), *Assessment and remediation of articulatory and phonological disorders* (pp. 355–359). Columbus, OH: Charles E. Merrill.

b. Overview

The Sensory-motor program was developed in the mid-1960s. It remains influential today largely because of its contention that the syllable is the basic unit of speech production (a controversial but popular idea) and because of the importance it places on phonetic environments in assessment and treatment. Treatment consists of production practice of treatment targets in various syllable contexts in increasingly complex levels of phonetic complexity. A client, for example, might be taught [t] before front vowels in nonsense CV syllables. Treatment might proceed to other vowel contexts, other syllable positions, and other speech levels, such as multisyllabic utterances. Practicing motor skills is believed by the authors to improve perceptual skills as well; therefore, perceptual training is not provided.

c. Comment

The emphasis that the Sensory-motor program placed on syllable and phonetic contexts foreshadowed later phonological approaches. The steps in a Sensory-motor program can be time-consuming to complete, and many clients are bored by its reliance on phonetic drills. Nonetheless, the program provides an option for use with more mature clients with intact cognitive skills.

4. Multiple Phoneme Program

a. References

McCabe, R., & Bradley, D. (1975). Systematic multiple phonemic approach to articulation therapy. *Acta Symbolica, 6,* 1–18.

Bradley, D. (1989). A systematic multiple-phoneme approach. In. N. Creaghead, P. Newman, & W. Secord (Eds.), *Assessment and remediation of articulatory and phonological disorders* (pp. 305–322). Columbus, OH: Charles E. Merrill.

b. Overview

The Multiple Phoneme program is a behaviorally oriented treatment method originally developed for children with repaired cleft palates. The Multiple Phoneme program is similar to the Van Riper method, with the major exception that, as its name implies, the Multiple Phoneme program allows more than one sound to be treated in a single treatment session. The authors place great emphasis on the need to collect ongoing data during treatment sessions.

c. Comments

The Multiple Phoneme program represents an early attempt to provide treatment to more than one sound at a time, an issue of primary importance for clients who have more severe articulation and phonological disorders. The program is rooted strongly in behaviorism and would be difficult to attempt without at least some acceptance of that theory. The program requires that the client know "letters" or phonetic symbols, which makes its use difficult with virtually all preschoolers. Finally, many younger school-age children find it confusing to receive treatment on more than one sound in a single treatment session.

5. Motoric Automatization of Articulatory Performance Program

a. Reference

Hoffman, P., Schuckers, G., & Daniloff, R. (1989). *Children's phonetic disorders: Theory and treatment.* Boston: Little, Brown.

b. Overview

This program (its somewhat cumbersome name is henceforth abbreviated MAP for Motoric Automatization Program) represents a recent attempt to provide treatment of speech problems from an articulation perspective. The primary goal of MAP is to provide practice in executing speech movements. This is achieved in two overlapping steps: stimulability and rehearsal. In the first step, the clinician elicits speech through imitation, which gives the client some experience of success as well as the opportunity to observe and imitate the clinician's demonstration. During this stage, the clinician also produces sounds with exaggeration (e.g., lots of lip rounding for labials) to give the client practice in manipulating the articulators in response to the clinician's model.

In the rehearsal step, the client practices treatment targets in increasingly complex linguistic levels and phonetic environments, including nonsense syllables, words and word pairs, sentences, and narratives. To help the client become aware of his or her speech errors, the clinician practices saying treatment targets as the client would. Other rehearsal activities include providing the client information on physiology and anatomy, viewing productions in a mirror, and listening to his or her speech on audio or video tapes.

c. Comment

MAP is an intelligent adaptation of an articulation approach to the treatment of clients with articulation and phonological disorders. As such, MAP offers a valuable treatment option for clients in Stage 4 with sufficient cognitive and attention abilities to reflect on their speech and to benefit from extensive motor practice.

B. Phonological Programs

Articulation approaches, which dominated the care of speech disorders for most of the 20th century, began to lose their appeal for many clinicians in the 1970s. The reason for this was that the primary tenets of articulation approaches — emphasis on individual sounds, phonetic drill, treatment of sounds in isolation and in nonsense syllables, improvements in small increments of change — although well suited to higher functioning clients with a few errors in late-acquired consonants and consonant clusters, proved far less useful with newer populations just appearing on the clinical horizon, many of whom were more severely involved preschoolers with speech problems affecting entire classes of sounds. Phonological approaches gained in popularity in the 1970s largely because their emphasis on sound as an aspect of language offered a means to treat the newer, more involved populations.

As indicated earlier in this chapter, currently two major types of phonological approaches exist: distinctive feature approaches (which attempt to encourage generalization based on the membership of sounds in sound classes) and phonological process approaches (which attempt to encourage generalization based on errors that classes of sounds undergo). Currently, the most influential distinctive feature program is that proposed by Blache (1989), and the most influential phonological process programs are the Cycles program, Metaphon, and Easy Does It For Phonology. An approach called contrast therapy is used in both some distinctive feature and phonological process programs. Contrast therapy activities are a loosely organized set of facilitative techniques rather than a treatment program, and they are discussed in Section IV (Word Pairs) in Chapter 5. Appendix 5B contains a relatively extensive list of word pairs for use in contrast therapy activities.

1. Blache's Distinctive Feature Program

a. Reference

Blache, S. (1989). A distinctive feature approach. In N. Creaghead, P. Newman, & W. Secord (Eds.), *Assessment and remediation of articulatory and phonological disorders* (pp. 361–382). Columbus, OH: Charles E. Merrill.

b. Overview

Distinctive feature approaches represented a first attempt to apply linguistic theory to the treatment of persons with articulation and phonological disorders. Early distinctive feature programs (Costello & Onstein, 1976; McReynolds & Engmann, 1975; McReynolds & Bennett, 1972) were actually hybrids of phonological and articulation approaches — the distinctive features used to promote generalization were phonological, and the activities used in treatment were motor-based. Although pioneering in their efforts and influential in their time, the first distinctive feature programs are no longer in wide use.

The most influential distinctive feature program today is Blache's (1989). In Blache's approach, sounds are taught as contrastive units within words using contrast therapy activities (see Chapter 5, Section IV). Treatment proceeds in four major steps. In Step 1, the clinician assesses the client's knowledge of the meanings of the words that are to be used in treatment. A client whose treatment target was [p], for example, might be shown pictures of a pan and a man, and asked, "Point to the one you use to cook. Point to the one that is another word for boy." In Step 2, the client is tested to determine if he or she can discriminate between word pairs differing by a single sound. A client, for example, might be shown the pictures of the pan and man, and asked to point the picture of the pan. In Step 3, the client is taught to distinguish between the word pairs in speech production. A client, for example, might be asked to say "pan," and the clinician then picks up the picture card that matches the client's pronunciation. To illustrate, if the client pronounced pan as man, the clinician would pick up the picture of the man. In Step 4, after the client can pronounce the treatment target at the word level, the word is placed in increasingly complex linguistic contexts, such as after a definite article, in three-word sentences, four-word sentences, and so on.

c. Comment

Blache's distinctive feature program represents the most recent attempt to apply distinctive feature theory to intervention with persons with speech problems. Blache's program (as well as the other distinctive feature programs cited above) utilizes distinctive features borrowed from linguistic theory rather than the familiar place, manner, and voicing distinctions used in this book and elsewhere (Williams, 1993). As several authors have observed, linguistic-based distinctive feature systems are intended to describe cross-language universals, and they are not always ideally suited to describing the speech of persons with articulation and phonological disorders (Folkins & Bleile, 1990; Parker, 1976). Blache's distinctive feature program is appropriate for selected clients in Stage 3 and clients in Stage 4.

2. Cycles Program

a. Reference

Hodson, B., & Paden, E. (1991). *Targeting intelligible speech.* Austin, TX: Pro-Ed.

b. Overview

The Cycles program is the most widely used phonological process approach in the United States. As its name suggests, the primary concept underlying this program is the cycle, which is a time period during which all error patterns that need remediation are facilitated in succession. Cycles last from 5 to 16 weeks, and, typically, three to six cycles (30–40 hours at 40–60 minutes per week) are usually required for a client to become intelligible. Error patterns are targeted for remediation based on percentage of occurrence (40% or greater), effect on intelligibility, and stimulability. Sounds in error patterns are selected for treatment based on stimulability. Typically, each sound in an error pattern receives 1 hour of therapy per cycle before the clinician goes on to the next sound in the error pattern. All error patterns targeted for remediation receive treatment in each cycle. Only one error pattern is targeted during a treatment session. Treatment activities consist of auditory bombardment, therapeutic play, and drill play to encourage production; probes to test for improvement and generalization; and a short home program for families.

c. Comment

Perhaps the most important insight of the Cycles program is its proposal that time rather than percentage correct is a better criterion for when to change treatment targets for most clients in Stage 2 and clients in Stage 3. The use of a time criterion appears to better replicate the gradual nature of articulation and phonological acquisition; a time criterion also appears better suited to the attention skills of a client in Stage 3 than does keeping a client on a task until a certain percentage criterion is obtained. Typically, the Cycles program does not utilize contrast therapy activities, although nothing in principle forbids doing so (Hodson, 1989). Tyler (1993) suggests that contrast therapy activities — whether as part of a Cycles program or as part of another approach — are more appropriate for clients who have relatively intact cognitive skills.

3. Metaphon Therapy

a. References

Dean, E., & Howell, J. (1986). Developing linguistic awareness: A theoretically based approach to phonological disorders. *British Journal of Disorders of Communication, 1,* 223–238.

Dean, E., Howell, J., Hill, A., & Waters, D. (1990). *Metaphon resource pack.* Windsor, UK: NFER-Nelson.

b. Overview

Metaphon therapy (metaphon is an abbreviation of metaphonology) was developed in the mid-1980s, and although Metaphon is not yet well known to most American speech-language clinicians, it has already found a receptive audience in Ireland and Great Britain. The primary tenet of Metaphon therapy is that phonological learning involves the client becoming aware of the contrastive nature of phonemes (Dean, Howell, Waters, & Reid, in press).

Metaphon therapy devotes great attention to teaching the client how to modify sounds to be more easily understood. Many activities used in Metaphon Therapy to achieve this result are already familiar to most speech-language clinicians, including the use of metaphors for sounds (e.g., [ʊ] might be called the "hissing sound") and contrast therapy activities. The most unique aspects of Metaphon are its heavy reliance on facilitative techniques to increase metalinguistic awareness and its tying of metalinguistics with a phonological approach. Another noteworthy aspect of Metaphon therapy is that it allows the client and clinician to negotiate the choice of metaphors to be used in treatment.

c. Comments

Metaphon therapy offers an interesting treatment option for clients in Stage 3 and Stage 4. The authors of Metaphon therapy have conducted a number of single-subject design experiments to test the effectiveness of their program and presently are engaged in a large-scale study to demonstrate its efficacy (Dean, Howell, & Waters, 1993).

4. Easy Does It for Phonology

a. Reference

Blodgett, E., & Miller, V. (1989). *Easy Does It For Phonology.*
East Moline, IL: LinguiSystems.

b. Overview

Easy Does It For Phonology (henceforth abbreviated EDIP)
is a relatively new program that combines aspects of several articulation, distinctive feature, and phonological
process approaches. The EDIP program consists of four
steps: (1) The client is bombarded with stimulus items so
he or she becomes aware of the distinctive feature being
omitted or distorted; (2) the client is taught that the presence or absence of a distinctive feature makes a difference in meaning; (3) the client learns to produce the target feature in various activities; and (4) the client learns to
produce the target feature and contrast it with his or her
phonological process. A very worthwhile contribution of
the authors is the development of simple metaphors to refer to consonant clusters, multisyllabic words, and word
positions (see Table 5–3).

c. Comment

EDIP offers a treatment option for clients in Stages 3 and
4 with relatively intact cognitive skills. EDIP combines
principles from articulation, distinctive feature, and phonological process approaches. EDIP's metaphors for
consonant clusters, multisyllabic words, and word positions are likely to find wide clinical use.

XIII. ASSESSMENT OF TREATMENT PROGRESS

Assessing the effectiveness of treatment is essential in managing
all clients, not least because periodic assessments of progress are
required by law, in most workplaces, and for reimbursement by insurance companies. The need for information on treatment outcome was listed as the highest health care priority by a recent
American Speech-Language-Hearing Association task force (Task
Force on Health Care, 1993). The two major options to assess treatment progress are pre- and post-tests and ongoing information
gathering.

Why Not Assess Progress Using Standardized Tests?

Standardized assessment instruments are seldom used to evaluate treatment progress, because the number of items that assess treatment targets is likely to be small. To illustrate, an assessment instrument testing 70 words is likely to contain only 3 or 4 words assessing [s], and only 1 of the words might assess [s] in word-initial position. If the clinician has spent a semester working on [s] in word-initial position, using the standardized assessment instrument will not show therapeutic gains.

A. Pre- and Post-tests

As the names suggest, pretests are administered prior to treatment (often as part of the assessment) and post-tests are administered at major junctures in treatment, often to determine if short- or long-term goals have been attained. Many clinicians, myself included, prefer pre- and post-tests to assess treatment progress, because they are quick and easy to administer and do not require attention to be directed away from the client during treatment sessions.

1. **Flexibility of Pre- and Post-tests.** Progress for any treatment target or treatment goal can be assessed using pre- and post-tests. A pre- and post-test for a client in Stage 1, for example, might assess the quantity or type of vocalizations produced during one or across several treatment sessions. Pre- and post-tests for a client in Stage 2, on the other hand, might assess the percentage of homonyms in the client's vocabulary or the number of sounds in the client's phonetic inventory. Similarly, a pre- and post-test for a client in Stage 3 might assess the percentage of occurrence of various error patterns, whereas a pre- and post-test for a client in Stage 4 might assess the percentage of correct productions of a sound on a picture naming task, or the number of correct productions of [sn] clusters in 1 minute of spontaneous speech describing a picture showing a "snow party." Results of pre- and post-tests are usually reported as percentage values. A possible statement in a clinical report is, "The client was administered pre- and post-tests of [s] in word-initial position. The client scored 20% correct in the pretest and 90% correct on the post-test."

2. **Examples.** Two quick and effective types of pre- and post-tests are word probes and judgment scales of severity and/or intelligibility. Many times a client receives both types of pre- and post-tests.

   a. **Word Probes.** The sound and error probes presented in Chapter 3 can easily be adapted into pre- and post-tests for clients in Stages 3 or 4. For example, a sound probe might indicate that a client was able to produce [s] 2 of 5 times word initially, and none of 5 times both between vowels and word-finally. This information could be used as the pretest, and the probe would be given again at the completion of treatment as the post-test. (There is no "correct" number of words that should be included in a probe. A general rule of thumb is 10 words per treatment target.) Error probes also can be used as pre-and post-tests. For example, the client might demonstrate a Fronting pattern on 8 of 10 words (80%) during the pretest and might demonstrate Fronting on 2 of 10 words (20%) on the post-test.

   b. **Intelligibility and Severity Testing.** Judgment scales of severity and intelligibility often serve as pre- and post-tests to assess treatment progress. Procedures to perform these measures were described in Chapter 3. If the judges are clinicians, three clinicians should be used, if possible. Clinical judgments of severity and intelligibility have the difficulties noted in Chapter 3, the chief of which is that the faster methods are highly subjective. Also, measures that show only a few degrees of disability may not be sufficiently sensitive to detect smaller increments of improvement. Results of intelligibility and severity judgment scales might be reported as, "Three of three trained speech-language clinicians judged the client to have a severe speech disorder before the onset of therapy. The client is now judged to have a mild speech disorder."

B. Ongoing Information Gathering

Although more time-consuming than pre- and post-tests, some clinicians collect ongoing information on the client's progress toward meeting a therapy objective. During each treatment session, for example, the clinician tabulates the client's rate of success, usually as a percentage value. To illustrate, the clinician might tabulate that the client is 50% accurate in producing a treatment target during session 1, 58% accurate in session 2, 64% accurate in session 3, and so on. Ongoing information gathering has an important advantage over pre- and post-testing in that it allows the clinician to more closely monitor the client's treatment progress.

Consumer Interviews

In addition to the assessments described in this section, treatment progress is always assessed by asking the client (when applicable), family, and significant persons in the client's environment if they have noticed change. The results should be included in the clinicial report.

C. Single-subject Design Experiments

Single-subject design experiments while a type of ongoing information gathering procedure, are sufficiently complex to warrant separate consideration.

Single-subject design experiments constitute an attempt to put clinical endeavors on a more rigorous scientific footing. Although commonly employed in behavioral psychology, single-subject design experiments have not found their way into widespread clinical use in speech-language pathology, perhaps because they are time-consuming to perform and their use requires some specialized knowledge. The information below outlines the basic steps and logic behind one type of single-subject design experiment, called a multiple baseline design. Before attempting such an experiment, the reader is referred to the more complete discussions on this topic appearing in McReynolds and Kearns (1983).

1. **Introduction.** Single-subject design experiments provide a method to demonstrate that improvement in the client results from the clinician's treatment, rather than from extraneous factors such as time and maturation.

2. **Multiple Baseline Design Experiments.** The type of single-subject design experiment that is most applicable to the clinical care of articulation and phonological disorders is called a multiple baseline design. A multiple baseline design can be used to evaluate treatment if (1) the client has at least two potential treatment targets and (2) the client's treatment targets are not so closely related that, when the client treats one target, the other target will also improve. For example, [p] and [b] would probably not be suitable treatment targets in a single-subject design experiment, because in many cases when a clinician focuses on [p] (or [b]) the cognate also improves. Better treatment targets for a single-subject design experiment might be [p] and [s], because improving one would not be expected to improve the other.

3. **Components of Multiple Baseline Design Experiments.** Multiple baseline design experiments consist of two phases, called A (baseline) and B (treatment). During the baseline, no treatment on the treatment target is provided. The baseline and treatment phases each must be at least three intervals (usually treatment sessions) in length. For example, data are collected during baseline for at least three treatment sessions, and treatment is provided for at least the same (and most likely more) number of sessions. Changes in percentage values between the baseline and treatment phases are the means most frequently used to demonstrate treatment progress. The results of the experiment are usually displayed as a simple graph of the type shown in Figure 4–1.

4. **Steps in Carrying Out a Multiple Baseline Experiment.** The following steps are used during a multiple baseline experiment.

   a. **Selection.** Select at least two treatment targets that are not so closely related that the client's progress in achieving one target is likely to affect the other target.

   b. **Baseline.** Begin collecting baseline data on both targets during the first session. For example, ask the client to pronounce 20 words beginning with the first treatment target and 20 different words beginning with the second treatment target. Graph the data as percentage of correct productions. Continue to collect baseline data for both treat-

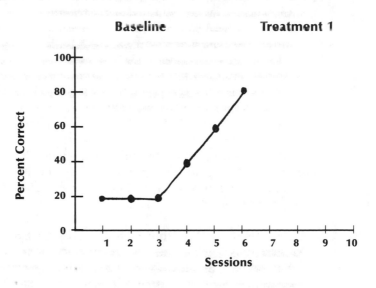

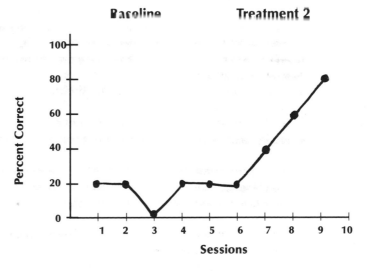

Figure 4-1. Example of a multiple basline experiment.

ment targets during at least three sessions. If the client begins to show improvement on the first treatment target prior to the end of baseline, continue collection of baseline data until the percentage of correct productions is the same for two sessions in a row or until the last session of baseline shows fewer correct productions than the session that preceded it. The purpose of collecting the additional baseline data is to ensure that improvement is not due to factors other than treatment. If the client continues to improve without treatment, the clinician should abandon the experiment because the client may not need treatment for that treatment target.

c. **Treatment (First Treatment Target).** Begin treatment for the first treatment target while continuing to collect baseline data for the second treatment target.

d. **Treatment (Second Treatment Target).** After criterion (typically 75% correct) is reached for the first target, begin treatment for the second treatment target. Continue to provide treatment for the second treatment target until criterion for it is reached as well.

CHAPTER

5

Facilitative Techniques

The following topics are discussed in this chapter:

I. OVERVIEW OF FACILITATIVE TECHNIQUES

The methods employed to effect change in a client's articulation and phonological development are called facilitative techniques. The term "facilitative" is usually preferred to "teaching" or "instruction" to emphasize that treatment is an interaction between the clinician's efforts and the client's capacity and willingness to learn. The major facilitative techniques employed in the treatment of articulation and phonological disorders include bombardment, metaphors, descriptions and demonstrations, touch cues, word pairs, building syllables and words, facilitative talk, and direct instruction.

II. BOMBARDMENT

Children typically acquire the sounds and syllables they hear more often. Bombardment is a well-established method used to increase the relative frequency of a treatment target in the client's environment (Nemoy & Davis, 1954). Typically, a client is not required to speak or vocalize during bombardment activities, only to listen. Some clinicians also recommend that the client wear a frequency modulated system during bombardment activities to increase the treatment target's saliency (Hodson, 1989). Depending on the client's age and the clinician's treatment philosophy, bombardment activities may last from a few minutes to 10 minutes. Some clinicians undertake bombardment only when introducing a new treatment target. Other clinicians include bombardment activities as part of each treatment session.

A. Stages 1 Through 3

Many clinicians begin each treatment session with clients in Stages 2 or 3 by bombarding the client with sounds, objects, and words containing the treatment target. (Bombardment might also be performed with clients in Stage 1, although it is not typical to do so.) Most commonly, the treatment target appears in the same position in all the words being used to bombard the client. Bombardment activities last from a few minutes up to approximately 10 minutes. A client in Stage 3 whose treatment target was [k], for example, might be exposed to objects beginning with [k] pulled out of a "magic box" or be asked to use a pretend fishing pole to "fish" objects out of a barrel. Typically, bombardment is followed by activities designed to stimulate production of the treatment target, although in principle it might also be provided without such a component. The most typical clinical situation in which a clinician might consider providing bombardment without a production component is as part of a stimulation program for clients in Stages 1 or 2 who are temporarily "stalled" in articulation and phonological development.

B. Stage 3 (Selected) and Stage 4

With more cognitively advanced clients in Stage 3 and clients in Stage 4, bombardment typically is used to introduce and later to prompt for treatment targets. The stimuli for bombardment activities often are specially designed stories or favorite stories containing frequent occurrences of the treatment target. A client, for example, might be instructed to "listen to a story in which the sound we're going to work on occurs lots of times." The client might also be instructed to ring a bell or raise his or her hand every time the sound occurs.

Metalinguistic Awareness

Metalinguistic awareness is the ability that allows persons to reflect on language. Techniques to facilitate metalinguistic awareness increase the client's awareness of short term goals and treatment targets. If, for example, the treatment target is [s], the clinician might label it "the long sound" to draw attention to a perceptual property (length) and place a paper in front of the client's mouth while saying [s] to draw attention to a production property (central air emission). Many activities traditionally called discrimination and perceptual training, although probably not "teaching" discrimination or perception, serve as valuable tools to facilitate metalinguistic awareness (Bleile & Hand, in press). Techniques particularly well-suited to facilitating metalinguistic awareness include metaphors, descriptions and demonstrations, touch cues, and word pairs.

III. METAPHORS, DESCRIPTIONS AND DEMONSTRATIONS, AND TOUCH CUES

Treatment generally proceeds more rapidly if the client is aware of the sounds and syllables that are the focus of remediation. The major techniques used to achieve this purpose are metaphors, descriptions and demonstrations, and touch cues, all of which are extremely useful when introducing new treatment targets, prompting, and promoting self-monitoring skills. Metaphors, descriptions and demonstrations, and touch cues for individual sounds are provided in Appendix 5A.

A. Metaphors

Metaphors compare some aspect of speech to something with which the client is familiar. A metaphor, for example, for [s] is "the snake sound," and a metaphor for a fricative is "the long sound." Possible metaphors for sound classes, syllables, and characteristics of words are listed in Tables 5-1, 5-2, and 5-3 (Blodgett & Miller, 1989; Flowers, 1990).

B. Descriptions and Demonstrations

Descriptions and demonstrations provide a simple means to heighten a client's awareness of selected characteristics of speech. A possible description of [p], for example, draws the client's attention to the closing lips, the build-up of air behind the lips, and the sudden release of air. A demonstration accompanying the description might involve placing a piece of paper in front of the client's lips to show the sudden release of air or gently pressing the client's lips together to show lip closure.

Table 5-1. Possible metaphors for places of production.

Place of Production	Metaphors
Bilabial	Lip sounds
Labiodental	Biting lip sounds or biting sounds
Interdental	Tongue tip sounds
Alveolar	Bump sounds, hill sounds
Postalveolar	Back of the hill sounds
Palatal	Middle sound
Velar	Back sounds
Glottal	Throat sound

Table 5-2. Possible metaphors for manners of production.

Manner of Production	Metaphors
Fricatives	Long sounds, hissing sounds
Glides and liquids (approximants)	Flowing sounds
Lateral	Side sound
Affricates	Engine chugging sounds
Nasals	Nose sounds
Stops	Short sounds, dripping sounds, and popping sounds
Voiced	Motor on, voice on, buzzing sound, hand buzzer sound, buzzing voice box, and voice box on
Voiceless	Motor off, voice off, not a buzzing sound, not a hand buzzer sound, no buzzing voice box, and voice box off

Table 5-3. Possible metaphors for consonant clusters, syllables, and words.

Sound Units	Metaphors
End of word	End sound
Multisyllabic words	Words with parts
Single syllable words	Words with one part
Initial consonants	Starting sounds
Consonant clusters	Sound friends

Source: Adapted from: *Easy Does It for Phonology* by E. Blodgett and V. Miller, 1989, East Moline, IL: LinguiSystems.

C. Touch Cues

Touch cues draw the client's attention to production characteristics of sounds (typically, the place of production). A client, for example, might be instructed to touch the lips for bilabial oral stops, to touch above the upper lip for alveolar stops, and to touch under the back of the chin for velar stops (Bleile & Hand, in press). Originally designed for clients with oral-motor dysfunction, touch cues are now finding their way into wider clinical use. Commonly used touch cues are listed in Table 5–4.

D. Stage 1

These techniques are not applicable with clients in Stage 1.

Table 5–4. Possible touch cues for place and manner of production.

Sound Class	Example		Touch Cue
Nasals	[m]		Fingers and thumb hold lips together; ask client to feel vibration on neck
	[n]		Lay finger over front of cheek bone
Oral Stops	[p]	[b]	Lay finger in front of lips
	[t]	[d]	Lay finger above top lip
	[k]	[g]	Lay finger at upper most part of neck
Fricatives	[f]	[v]	Lay finger below bottom lip
	[θ]	[ð]	Place finger in front of lips and remind client to protrude tongue
	[s]		Point to the corner of the mouth (to indicate spread) and remind client of the teeth being together
	[ʃ]		Lay finger in front of lips and use the metaphor "quiet sound"
Liquid	[l]		Lay tip of finger on middle of upper lip
Diphthongs	[oʊ]		Trace with finger around lips and use the metaphor "blowing sound"
	[eɪ]		Lay fingers on corners of mouth and use the metaphor "smiling sound"

E. Stage 2

Metaphors, descriptions, and demonstrations are generally not effective with clients in Stage 2. Interestingly, however, some clients in Stage 2 respond well to touch cues even though they may lack the cognitive maturation required to identify places of production. Perhaps touch cues are effective with these clients because they prompt the client to produce a sound in a way that the clinician praises rather than because the cues help the client focus on a particular place of production (Bleile & Hand, in press).

F. Stage 3

Touch cues are effective with almost all clients in Stage 3. Metaphors are effective with most clients, and descriptions and demonstrations are effective with more cognitively advanced clients.

As with clients in Stage 2, touch cues are introduced early in treatment. Metaphors for treatment targets are also introduced early in the course of treatment, preferably through negotiation with the client (Dean et al., 1990). After the metaphor is established, practice is provided to help the client associate the metaphor with the treatment target. If, for example, the treatment target is [s], the clinician might ask the client, "Raise your hand when I say our snake sound. Is it [ʃ]? Is it [f]? Is it [s]?" If the client experiences difficulty associating the metaphor with the treatment target, the number of features distinguishing the treatment target from the other sounds is increased. For example, if the client in the above example raised his or her hand for [f], the clinician might then contrast [s] with [l] or with vowels. Metaphors also provide a valuable means to prompt productions and to facilitate self-monitoring skills during the course of treatment. For example, if the client says [t] for [s], the client might be asked, "Was that the snake sound?"

Trial use of descriptions and demonstrations should be attempted early in treatment with more developmentally advanced clients. If the client appears unable to comprehend or benefit from this facilitative technique, the clinician should place greater reliance on touch cues and metaphors.

G. Stage 4

Metaphors, descriptions and demonstrations, and touch cues are effective with clients in Stage 4. Touch cues and metaphors may be used with less advanced clients in this stage, although care is needed to ensure that the client does not feel he or she is being treated "like a baby." Descriptions and demonstrations are valuable with clients in Stage 4 who have sufficient cognitive and attention abilities to comprehend the instructions used in these tasks. Clients with limited cognitive and attention skills who find descriptions and demonstrations confusing may benefit from treatment that makes greater use of metaphors.

Special Words

In treatment all words are not equal. Words that the client considers important to pronounce often provide the best focus for treatment activities. Treatment, for example, might focus on names of favorite objects and persons that contain the treatment target or specific words that are pronounced in such a way as to provoke teasing. Treatment with more advanced clients in Stage 4 might focus on multisyllable words that appear in school or work assignments.

IV. WORD PAIRS

Languages use sound to distinguish the meaning of words. The difference in meaning between "cup" and "pup," for example, is that the former begins with [k] and the latter with [p]. The contrastive nature of sound is used to facilitate perception and production through word pairs (also called minimal and maximal pairs) that differ by a single sound (Elbert, Rockman, & Saltzman, 1982; Tyler, Edwards, & Saxman, 1987; Weiner, 1981). The words "bee-pea," for example, are a word pair in which the words differ from each other by one sound, [b] and [p]. The words "bee" and "pea" are a minimal pair, because they differ by a single distinctive feature (voicing) in most distinctive feature systems. Word pairs can also differ by more than one distinctive feature (called maximal pairs), as in "pea-me," which differ in voicing ([p] is voiceless and [m] is voiced) and nasality ([p] is an oral consonant and [m] is a nasal consonant).

Some evidence suggests that use of maximal pairs is more effective with clients in the early stages of articulation and phonological development, and that minimal pairs may be more appropriate for clients in later stages of articulation and phonological development (Gierut, 1989). Word pairs may also differ in the presence or absence of a sound, such as in "bee-beet" and "slow-low." Lists of word pairs for word-initial consonants, word-initial consonant cluster reduction, word-final consonants, and word-final consonant deletion are provided in Appendix 5B (Walsh, 1994).

A. Stages 1 Through 3

Word pairs are not applicable for use with clients in Stage 1 and Stage 2. Nor are they useful with less cognitively advanced clients in Stage 3.

B. Stage 3 (Selected) and Stage 4

The greatest utility of word pairs is with more cognitively advanced clients in Stage 3 and clients in Stage 4.

1. **Perception.** Word pairs are used in contrast therapy activities to facilitate perception of newly introduced treatment targets (Elbert, Rockman, & Saltzman, 1980; Weiner, 1981). Typically, words containing the treatment target are contrasted with words containing the client's error. For example, a client whose treatment target was [p] and who pronounced [p] as [b] word-initially might be shown a picture of a pea and a bee, and be instructed, "I am going to show you two pictures. You point to the one I say. Bee. Good. Now point to pea. Good." Most commonly, 5 to 10 word pairs are presented in this manner with the clinician alternating whether the treatment target is the first or second member of the pair.

   If the client experiences difficulty with the above task, real objects might be used in place of pictures, or the treatment target might be contrasted with a nonerror sound (e.g., "bee-see" for the client in the example). Reminding the client of a metaphor for the treatment target may also assist in this task. If the client is somewhat older, a list of words might be used instead of pictures or objects. In this situation, the client would be instructed, "I'm going to say two words. You tell me if the words sound the same or different. Ready? Pea-bee. Are they the same or different?"

2. **Production.** Word pairs are also used in contrast therapy activities as a preferred means to facilitate speech production (Elbert, Rockman, & Saltzman, 1980; Weiner, 1981). As was the case in facilitating perception, the client is presented with word pairs contrasting the treatment target with the client's error. The client discussed above, for example, might be presented a picture of a pea and a bee and be asked, "Tell me which one grows in the ground." If the client says [bi], he or she is given the picture of the bee, and the clinician explains, "But you said bee." As above, 5 to 10 word pairs are typically presented in this manner and the clinician occasionally presents word pairs the client can produce correctly, so he or she will not become discouraged. If the client experiences difficulty with this task, real objects may be used in place of pictures. Reminding the client of a metaphor for the treatment target often proves helpful, as does a description or demonstration of the treatment target.

V. BUILDING SYLLABLES AND WORDS

Most facilitative techniques target sounds rather than syllables and words. The metaphors described in Tables 5-1 and 5-2, for example, describe sound classes, whereas the metaphors, descriptions and demonstrations, and touch cues appearing in Appendix 5A focus on individual sounds. The information provided in Table 5-3 represents a step in the development of a vocabulary with which to talk to clients directly about syllables and words. Bernhardt (in press) has pioneered efforts to develop techniques to facilitate syllable and word development. Three specific techniques focus on final consonants, consonant clusters, and retention of syllables.

Beyond the Isolated Word

Many of the elicitation activities described in Chapter 2 help a client move from isolated words to phrases, sentences, and spontaneous speech. Other activities include:

Read a story whose main characters and actions contain the treatment target. Then ask the client to tell you the story.

Play a game in which the client tells a story containing characters whose names contain the treatment target. For younger clients, it sometimes helps to let the client hold a puppet that tells the story.

Take turns with the client telling a story in which the names of characters and actions contain the treatment target. The length of turns in the game can be phrases, sentences, or episodes.

Play a barrier game in which the names of the objects contain the treatment target.

For more mature clients, ask the client to make up phrases, sentences or short stories containing the treatment target.

A. Final Consonants

Many clients experience difficulty in using consonants to close syllables and words. A client, for example, might pronounce "beet" as [bi] through Final Consonant Deletion. Bernhardt recommends using a rhyming word task to remediate this error pattern (Bernhardt, in press). In this task, a client is first presented a story containing rhyming words ending in vowels. Once the client appears to grasp the concept of rhymes, rhyming words ending in consonants are introduced. The first story, for example, might involve "Pooh," "Roo," and cows that go "moo," while the second story (or continuation of the first story) might involve a girl named "June" who sings a "tune" to the "moon" while standing on a "dune."

B. Consonant Clusters

The acquisition of consonant clusters often presents a significant difficulty to clients. A client, for example, might pronounce "ski" as [ki] through Cluster Reduction. The remediation principle used to facilitate consonant cluster development is the same one that causes speakers to typically pronounce "is" as "tis" in phrases such as "It is" (Bleile, 1991b). In such phrases, the final consonant ([t] in this case) tends to migrate to the following syllable if that syllable begins with a vowel. Similarly, a consonant cluster can be introduced into word-initial position through phrases such as "ask a," which, if said quickly, is likely to be pronounced as "a ska" (Bernhardt, in press).

C. Retention of Syllables

Even after a client is able to produce most sounds, he or she may still experience difficulty retaining unstressed syllables in longer words, words with unusual stress patterns, and word compounds. A client, for example, might be able to say "in," but may delete the same syllable when it occurs in a word such as "serendipity" through a developmentally advanced form of Syllable Deletion.

Remediation to retain syllables is accomplished in three steps (Bernhardt, in press). First, the client practices multisyllabic words, producing them with equal syllable intensities and durations. Next, the client is provided practice in alternating loud-soft and short-long syllables. Third, the client is taught to use key words and rhythm cues. The STRONG-weak-STRONG stress pattern, for example, might be called "the elephant's beat," and the weak-STRONG-weak stress pattern might be called "Aladdin's beat." (Capital letters indicate primary stress.) A possible variation on this procedure is to use visual and tactile cues to illustrate the number of syllables in a word. A clinician, for example, might have the client place a bead on a string for every syllable in the word. A Hawaiian variation on this activity is to let the beads represent flowers on a lei (Imanaka-Inouye, 1994, personal communication).

D. Stages 1 and 2

Clients in Stages 1 and 2 lack the prerequisite cognitive abilities to perform these treatment tasks.

E. Stage 3 (Selected) and Stage 4

These tasks are appropriate for clients in Stage 3 who have more cognitively advanced abilities and for clients in Stage 4 without major intellectual disabilities, cognitive impairments, or limitations in attention. The word pairs for Consonant Final Deletion (Appendix 5B) can serve as a source of rhyming words, which can then be presented as a list or, more interestingly, in a story format. To help facilitate perception, the client might be asked to ring a bell or raise his or her hand whenever a rhyme is heard. For example, the client might be instructed: "Raise your hand every time you hear a word that rhymes with Pooh." To facilitate production, the client might be taught to recite an entertaining short story containing the rhyming words.

Activities for consonant clusters might include "talking over" games. A client, for example, might be instructed to "say this over and over again: 'ask a.' " The client would then say, "askaaskaaska," until "a ska" results. The client would then be instructed to throw away or drop the initial "a," resulting in "ska." The syllable "ska" might then be used as the basis from which to generalize [sk] clusters to word-initial environments. The same general technique might also be used to help facilitate word-initial consonants in clients whose speech contains Initial Consonant Deletion.

Any number of activities might be developed to facilitate retention of syllables, ranging from drills to elaborate games and stories. For example, a game could be made of saying all difficult multisyllabic words on a homework assignment with equal stress. Next, a game could be made of saying the words with exaggerated stress patterns, saying the unstressed syllables very slowly and the stressed syllables very loudly. An additional tactile cue is to play a game in which the client claps his or her hands on the stressed syllables (or slaps his or her desktop). Alternately, if the client experiences difficulty producing the most heavily stressed syllable in the word, hand clapping might be reserved for that syllable. Finally, key words are often crucial to treatment success in facilitating stress patterns. The best words for this purpose are those of well-liked animals (e.g., elephant and buffalo for STRONG-weak-strong stress patterns), cartoon characters, and, for older clients, words likely to arise in the course of school assignments.

VI. FACILITATIVE TALK

Facilitative talk is a body of techniques for talking with clients who have articulation and phonological disorders and language disorders (Bleile, in press). For some clients, facilitative talk is an adjunct to more direct instruction; for others, it is the primary means of intervention. The principle options for facilitative talk include motherese, repetitions, strategic errors, modeling, parallel talk, and requests for confirmation or clarification. Motherese is used with clients in Stage

1, and the other types of facilitative talk are used with clients in later stages. Many of the assessment activities described in Chapter 2 provide excellent venues for facilitative talk.

The Comfort Zone

Infants tend to vocalize most when they are in the comfort zone — an emotional state in which they feel secure, safe, and contented. Rapport and knowledge of an infant's likes and daily routines are far more likely to stimulate infant vocalizations than reliance on any particular facilitative technique or elicitation activity. This is why parents are more likely to facilitate their children's vocalizations than clinicians. When a parent is not available or is unable to perform this task, however, the clinician can perform it successfully — if the infant likes the clinician and the clinician knows the infant well.

A. Motherese

Motherese is a combination of facilitative talk techniques that serve to capture and keep an infant's attention (Dore, 1986; Snow, 1984). Motherese speech modifications include:

Higher than usual pitch

Talking about shared perceptions

Exaggerated intonation

Use of repetitions

Calling attention to objects

Imitation games can be used in conjunction with motherese. Infants as young as 1 month of age are occasionally able to imitate vocalizations they already produce, and near 8 months of age most infants will occasionally imitate new types of vocalizations.

B. Expansions

Expansions "fill in the incorrect or missing speech parts." The client, for example, might say [pi] for "bee," and the clinician might repeat the word, changing [p] to [b]. Alternately, if the client deleted [t] in "beet," the clinician might repeat the client, expanding [bi] to [bit].

C. Strategic Errors

Strategic errors are clinician-produced speech errors that mimic aspects of the client's articulation and phonological disorder. If, for example, the client pronounced word-initial [t] as [d], during the course of play the clinician might point to a doll's toe and say, "Doe." The hoped-for response is for the client to look confused or laugh and then attempt to say the word with an initial [t].

D. Modeling

Modeling involves the use of the clinician, another person, or a favored toy as a speech example. In a modeling game, for example, the clinician might introduce a puppet as the teacher and the client and clinician as the students. The puppet teacher instructs the students to repeat what she says, which are words that contain the treatment target.

E. Parallel Talk

In parallel talk the clinician talks about the client's actions and the objects to which he or she is attending. For example, with a client who has [b] as a treatment target, the clinician might fill the clinic room with objects containing this sound. When the client looks at a ball, the clinician might say "ball," and as the client rolls the ball across the floor, the clinician might say, "Ball rolling" or "Here comes the ball."

F. Requests for Confirmation or Clarification

Requests for confirmation or clarification are techniques designed to focus the client's attention on the communicative adequacy of his or her speech. During play, for example, a client whose treatment target was [k] might say "key" as "tea." The clinician might ask, "Did you say tea?" or "What did you say you wanted?" or "Did you say you wanted some tea?" or "I thought I heard you say tea. Is that what you meant to say?" The hoped-for response is that the client will repeat, "key" or say something like, "I said key."

Baby Talk

Families frequently ask clinicians whether or not to use "baby talk" with young children. Family members should talk to their children in ways that are fun for the children and enjoyable and natural for the caregiver (Bleile, 1991a; Silverman, McGowan, Bleile, Fus, & Barnas, 1993). A child who has fun communicating is more likely to want to do it again. Caregivers might be counseled to keep the following questions in mind when interacting with a young child: Does the child appear interested? Is the child paying attention? Caregivers should speak in whatever way maximizes the chance that they can answer "yes" to both of these questions. For most children, "yes" answers are achieved most often if adults use simple language. Simplifying language means using short sentences and single words, talking about the "here and now," and talking about what appears to interest the child. For example, if the child appears interested in a stuffed animal, a caregiver might say, "Teddy Bear." Next, the caregiver might pet the stuff animal, saying, "Soft," and then give the bear to the child to pet.

G. Stage 1

The primary facilitative talk technique used with clients in Stage 1 is motherese. Many investigators believe that routines provide the predictability in words and actions that facilitate the acquisition of speech and language (Bruner, 1983; Snow & Goldfield, 1983). For this reason, intervention with clients in Stage 1 typically begins with establishing routines between the client and the clinician (or caregiver). Possible routines include daily activities involving mealtime, diaper changing, and dressing, or "my turn your turn" games such as "peek-a-boo" and "so big." Stimulation of vocal development then proceeds in the context of these shared routines (Bleile, in press).

Some clients in Stage 1 can be encouraged to vocalize through reciprocal communication games based on imitation. For example, the client says [bi] during play, and the clinician says [bi] in response, and the client then imitates the clinician. A more adult-centered variation of this game is for the clinician to introduce the vocalization that serves as the basis of the reciprocal communication. For example, the clinician says [di di] for the client to imitate. Reciprocal communiction games are also used to stimulate more developmentally advanced types of vocalizations. For example, the client says [di di] (reduplicated babbling), and the clinician then says [di bi] (nonreduplicated babbling) for the client to imitate.

The Silent Infant

Vocal development can proceed even if an infant is temporarily unable to vocalize due to medical or physical reasons. In such situations, the infant can still learn about the perceptual and communicative value of sound from interacting with others. The infant's contribution to such dialogues may include eye widening, smiling, movement of the extremities, or imitative oral motor movements. Even if a child will not ever have the ability to vocalize, engaging in reciprocal communication is still valuable in promoting social and language development.

H. Stage 2

The primary facilitative talk techniques used with clients in Stage 2 are expansions, requests for confirmation or clarification, modeling, and parallel talk. Expansions are useful in helping the client perceive the contrast between the client's and the clinician's speech, as well as in providing an example for the client to reproduce. Requests for confirmation or clarification (e.g., asking "What did you say" or "I don't understand") help the client focus on the adequacy of his or her speech as a means of communication.

Modeling and parallel talk, in addition to offering the client perceptual information about the use of sounds in words, also may facilitate production as the client repeats the words spoken by the clinician. Most often, the speech model is the clinician or a family member, although some clients can also play simple versions of modeling games in which the model is a favorite stuffed animal or doll. In addition to the above techniques, a few clients in Stage 2 also respond appropriately to strategic errors, although most simply look confused and continue what they are doing.

I. Stage 3

All of the facilitative talk techniques used with clients in Stage 2 are also ideally suited to the interests and cognitive development of clients in Stage 3.

1. **Expansions and Parallel Talk.** As with clients in Stage 2, expansions and parallel talk expose the client to opportunities to perceive and produce speech.

2. **Strategic Errors.** Strategic errors are useful as a technique to help the client both identify his or her articulation and phonological errors and produce treatment targets.

3. **Modeling.** Modeling is a particularly useful technique to facilitate the production of treatment targets. For example, the client's speech might contain a Prevocalic Voicing pattern, and the treatment target might be [t] in the word-initial position. In one activity, a puppet might recite a list of her favorite words, sometimes pronouncing word-initial [t] as [d] and other times pronouncing it correctly. The client's role is to tell the puppet when she says the word correctly. In an alternate modeling activity, the puppet might be the teacher and the client's role is to repeat what the teacher says, thus facilitating speech production.

4. **Requests for Confirmation or Clarification.** Requests for confirmation or clarification are useful in facilitating the client's identification and production of treatment targets. During a game, for example, the client described above might pronounce "team" as "deem." The clinician might then ask, "I didn't understand you — what did you say?" or "Did you say you want to play on the deem?"

J. Stage 4

Although treatment with clients in Stage 4 typically involves direct instruction, treatment can also use modified versions of strategic errors, modeling, and requests for confirmation or clarification. To illustrate, suppose a client's treatment target is word-initial [s]. When providing strategic errors, the clinician might read a story, sometimes pronouncing word-initial [s] with a frontal lisp and other times pronouncing it correctly. The client's role is to identify when an error is produced. The same activity can be altered into a speech production activity by having the client identify and correct any instances in which [s] is pronounced as a frontal lisp.

A possible modeling activity for clients in Stage 4 is to have the clinician read a word or sentence containing the treatment target and then to say the same utterance exactly as the clinician did. A possible request for confirmation or clarification activity is to instruct the client to speak on a topic of interest. The clinician then stops the client and asks for confirmation or clarification each time a treatment target is pronounced incorrectly.

VII. DIRECT INSTRUCTION: PHONETIC PLACEMENT AND SHAPING TECHNIQUES

Phonetic placement and shaping techniques were the stock-and-trade of speech-language clinicians for much of the 20th century (Fairbanks, 1960; Nemoy & Davis, 1954). The use and knowledge of these techniques has declined in recent years, because client populations have shifted downward in age and increased in severity of involvement. Still, many clients benefit from careful use of phonetic placement and shaping techniques, especially with more cognitively advanced clients in Stage 3 and most clients in Stage 4.

Imitation

Imitation is used as a direct instruction technique with some clients in Stage 2, most clients in Stage 3, and almost all clients in Stage 4. A clinician, for example, might ask a client to imitate a treatment target when introducing a new treatment target and periodically during treatment "to remind" the client of the correct production.

A. Phonetic Placement

Phonetic placement techniques teach the tongue and lip positions used in speech production. Phonetic placement techniques to teach [t], for example, ask the client to raise the tongue tip, touch the tongue tip to the alveolar ridge, and to quickly draw the tongue tip down again. Phonetic placement techniques for American English consonants and [ɚ] are provided in Appendix 5C.

B. Shaping

Shaping techniques use a sound the client can already produce (either a speech error or another sound) to learn a new sound. Shaping techniques, for example, provide a series of steps through which a client who says [w] is taught to say [r]. Shaping techniques for American English consonants and [ɚ] are provided in Appendix 5C.

C. Stages 1 Through 3

Direct instruction techniques are not applicable for use with clients in Stages 1 and 2 or with most clients in Stage 3.

D. Stage 3 (Selected) and Stage 4

Phonetic placement and shaping techniques are sometimes useful with more cognitively advanced clients in Stage 3 and with attentive clients in Stage 4.

Phonetic placement and shaping techniques are guidelines rather than rigid procedures. The clinician should pick and choose among treatment techniques, keeping what works, discarding what does not, and (most often) modifying a technique to better suit the clinician's style and the client's needs. The activities used to teach phonetic placement and shaping techniques are limited only by the clinician's imagination. Place of production for alveolar stops, for example, might be indicated using peanut butter or by instructing the client to use his or her tongue tip to "touch the hill on the top of your mouth." Similarly, the release of air occurring during release of a stop might be indicated by placing a hand, a piece of paper, or a paper flower in front of the client's mouth.

Appendix 5A

Metaphors, Descriptions and Demonstrations, and Touch Cues

A. Introduction

Options for metaphors, descriptions and demonstrations, and touch cues for consonants and [ɚ] are listed in this appendix. Rather than list a voiced and voiceless demonstration for each pair of obstruents, ideas for demonstrating this contrast are listed in Table 5–5.

Table 5–5. Five possible methods to demonstrate voicing.

Methods	Instructions
1.	Instruct the client to listen to and identify the difference between a voiceless and voiced [ɑ].
2.	Place the client's hands over the ears and instruct him or her to hum, which heightens the sensation of vocal cord vibration.
3.	If the client is able to produce a voiced and voiceless fricative, ask him or her to cover the ears and make these sounds. Alternatively, ask the client to make [h] and [ɑ].
4.	You and the client place one hand on your throat and the other on the client's throat while making voiced and voiceless sounds together. Tell each other when the voicing goes on and off.
5.	If the client is able to produce a voiced and voiceless oral stop, attach a small piece of paper or a paper flower to the end of a tongue depressor or pencil and ask the client to "make the paper (or flower) move." The paper is more likely to move when a voiceless consonant is produced than when a voiced consonant is produced. (Be careful in providing instructions to the client, however, because a strongly articulated voiced oral stop will also move the flower.)

[p] and [b]

DESCRIPTION: Draw attention to closing the two lips, the build-up of pressure behind the lips, and the sudden release of air through the mouth. For [b], also draw attention to the buzzing voice box.

METAPHORS: [p] is the popping sound and the sound beginning "pop," "pie," and "pig." [b] is the bubble sound and the sound beginning "bye," "bee," and "bed." [p] and [b] are also short sounds (stops) and lip sounds (bilabials). Additionally, [b] is made with the motor on (voiced).

TOUCH CUE: Place the client's finger in front of his or her lips.

DEMONSTRATIONS:

Place (Bilabial)

First Method: Lightly touch the client's upper and lower lips with a tongue depressor, then ask the client to bring the lips together to touch the spot you touched.

Second Method: Ask the client to make kissing noises.

Manner (Oral Stop)

First Method: Use a strip of paper, a feather, or the hand held in front of the client's mouth while you produce a series of stops to demonstrate the explosive release of stops. Alternately, tape a small paper flower on the end of a pencil and encourage the client to move the flower with puffs of air.

Second Method: Place your or the client's palms together and then suddenly separate them to demonstrate the sudden release of stops.

[m]

DESCRIPTION: Draw attention to closing the lips, the build up of pressure behind the lips, the buzzing in the throat, and the outward flow of air through the nose.

METAPHORS: The humming sound and the sound beginning "mom," "moo," and "me." [m] is also a motor-on sound (voiced), a nose sound (nasal), and a lip sound (bilabial).

TOUCH CUE: Use the client's fingers and thumb to hold his or her lips together.

DEMONSTRATIONS:

Place (Bilabial)

First Method: Lightly touch the client's upper and lower lips with a tongue depressor, then ask the client to bring the lips together to touch the spot you touched.

Second Method. Ask the client to make kissing noises.

Manner (Nasal Stop)

First Method: Contrast breathing through the nose onto a mirror or piece of paper with breathing through the mouth onto a mirror or piece of paper.

Second Method: Instruct the client to take deep breath, hold it, and let air out through the nose to produce a voiceless nasal sound.

Third Method: To demonstrate nasality with voicing, instruct the client to take a deep breath, hold it, and say "ah" with the mouth closed so air comes out the nose. Telling the client to open his or her mouth will help teach release of a nasal consonant.

[w]

DESCRIPTION: The round lip sound or the wow sound (wow!) and the sound that begins "wow," "we," and "why." [w] is also a lip sound (bilabial), a back sound (velar), and a buzzing sound (voiced).

TOUCH CUES: None.

DEMONSTRATIONS:

Place (Bilabial)

First Method: Lightly touch the client's upper and lower lips with a tongue depressor, then ask the client to bring the lips together to touch the spot you touched.

Second Method: Ask the client to make kissing noises.

Manner (Approximant)

First Method: Use a strip of paper, a feather, or the hand held in front of the client's mouth while you produce several glides or liquids to draw attention to the "flowing" quality and continuous nature of the sounds. Alternately, tape a small paper flower on the end of a pencil and encourage the client to move the flower in the wind.

Second Method: Run your or the client's finger down the client's arm while making several long glides or liquids to demonstrate the "flowing" quality and length of these sounds.

[f] and [v]

DESCRIPTION: Draw attention to the lower lip touching the upper teeth and the outward flowing of air from the mouth. For [v], also draw attention to the motor being on.

METAPHORS: [f] is the angry cat sound ("ffff") and the sound beginning "feet," "fun," or "fish." [v] is the jet sound, the sound beginning "very," "volcano," and "vanilla." [f] and [v] are also long sounds (fricatives) and tooth sounds (labiodental). [v] is made with the motor on (voiced).

TOUCH CUE: Lay the client's finger below his or her bottom lip.

DEMONSTRATIONS:

Place (Labiodental)

First Method: Lightly touch the client's lower lip and the bottom of the upper front teeth with a tongue depressor, then ask the client to bring the upper teeth and lower lip together to touch where you touched.

Second Method: Ask the client to bite his or her lower lip gently with his upper teeth.

Manner (Fricative)

First Method: Use a strip of paper, a feather, or the hand held in front of the client's mouth while you produce several long voiceless fricatives to draw attention to the "hissing" quality and continuous nature of the sounds. An alternate method is to tape a small paper flower on the end of a pencil and encourage the client to move the flower in the wind.

Second Method: Run your or the client's finger down the client's arm while making several long voiceless fricatives to demonstrate the "hissing" quality and length of fricatives.

[θ] and [ð]

DESCRIPTION: Draw attention to the tongue tip between the upper and lower front teeth. For [ð], also draw attention to the buzzing voice box.

METAPHORS: [θ] is the leaking tire sound. [ð] is the motor-on sound. [θ] and [ð] are also long sounds (fricative) and tongue-teeth sounds (interdental). [ð] is also made with the voice on (voiced).

TOUCH CUE: Place the client's finger in front of his or her lips and remind the client to extrude his or her tongue.

DEMONSTRATIONS:

Place (Interdental)

First Method: Ask the client to stick the tongue out and then gently close his or her mouth (if the tongue is sticking out too far, push it back with a tongue depressor).

Second Method: Place a tongue depressor or piece of food in front of the client's mouth, ask the client to touch it with the tongue, and then to close the mouth gently.

Manner (Fricative)

First Method: Use a strip of paper, a feather, or the hand held in front of the mouth while you produce several long voiceless fricatives to draw attention to the "hissing" quality and continuous nature of the sounds. An alternate method is to tape a small paper flower on the end of a pencil and encourage the client to move the flower in the wind.

Second Method: Run your or the client's finger down the client's arm while making several long voiceless fricatives to demonstrate the "hissing" quality and length of fricatives.

[t] and [d]

DESCRIPTION: Draw attention to the tongue tip touching the bump behind the upper front teeth. For [d], also draw attention to the motor being on.

METAPHORS: [t] is the tick-tock sound and the sound that begins "toe," "tummy," and "Tommy." [d] is the do sound ("I can do it") or the Homer Simpson sound (Doh!), and the sound that begins "dinner," "doll," and "done." [t] and [d] are also tongue tip sounds (alveolar) and short sounds (stop). [d] is made with the voice on (voiced).

TOUCH CUE: Lay the client's finger above his or her upper lip.

DEMONSTRATIONS:

Place (Alveolar)

First Method: Ask the client to feel the bump on the roof of his or her mouth just behind the two front teeth.

Second Method: Place a little peanut butter or a favored food on a Q-tip, touch the Q-tip to the alveolar ridge, and ask the client to remove the food with the tongue tip.

Manner (Oral Stop)

First Method: Use a strip of paper, a feather, or the hand held in front of the client's mouth while you produce a series of stops to demonstrate the explosive release of stops. Alternately, tape a small paper flower on the end of a pencil and encourage the client to move the flower with puffs of air.

Second Method: Place your or the client's palms together and then suddenly separate them to demonstrate the sudden release of stops.

[n]

DESCRIPTION: Draw attention to the tongue tip touching the bump behind the upper front teeth, the buzzing in the voice box, and the air coming out through the nose.

METAPHORS: The siren sound and the first sound in "no," "knee," and "night." [n] is also a nose sound (nasal) and a tongue tip sound (alveolar).

TOUCH CUE: Lay the client's finger over the front of his or her cheek bone.

DEMONSTRATIONS:

Place (Alveolar)

First Method: Ask the client to feel the bump on the roof of his or her mouth just behind the two front teeth.

Second Method: Place a little peanut butter or a favored food on a Q-tip, touch the Q-tip to the alveolar ridge, and ask the client to remove the food with the tongue tip.

Manner (Nasal Stop)

First Method: Contrast breathing through the nose onto a mirror or piece of paper with breathing through the mouth onto a mirror or piece of paper.

Second Method: Instruct the client to take a deep breath, hold it, and let air out through the nose to produce a voiceless nasal sound.

Third Method: To demonstrate nasality with voicing, instruct the client to take a deep breath, hold it, and say "ah" with the mouth closed so that air comes out the nose. Telling the client to open the mouth will help teach release of a nasal consonant.

[s] and [z]

DESCRIPTION: Draw attention to the hissing sound and the position of the tongue tip (behind the front upper or lower teeth). For [z], also draw attention to the buzzing voice box.

METAPHORS: [s] is the snake sound or the hissing sound and the sound that begins "sun," "sit," and "Santa." [z] is the bee sound and the sound that begins "zoo," "zero," and "zebra." [s] and [z] are also long sounds (fricative) and tongue tip sounds (alveolar). [z] is made with the voice on (voiced).

TOUCH CUE: None. These sounds are usually acquired too late in development for the touch cue technique to be appropriate.

DEMONSTRATIONS:

Place (Alveolar)

First Method: Ask the client to feel the bump on the roof of his or her mouth just behind the two front teeth.

Second Method: Place a little peanut butter or a favored food on a Q-tip, touch the Q-tip to the alveolar ridge, and ask the client to remove the food with the tongue tip.

Manner (Fricative)

First Method: Use a strip of paper, a feather, or the hand held in front of the client's mouth while you produce several long voiceless fricatives to draw attention to the "hissing" quality and continuous nature of the sounds. Alternately, tape a small paper flower on the end of a pencil and encourage the client to move the flower in the wind.

Second Method: Run your or the client's finger down the client's arm while making several long voiceless fricatives to demonstrate the "hissing" quality and length of fricatives.

[l]

DESCRIPTION: Draw attention to the tongue tip raised to the mouth roof, the air flowing over the sides of the tongue, and the buzzing of the voice box.

METAPHORS: The singing sound (la-la-la) or the pointy sound (i.e., the tongue is pointing at the alveolar ridge), and the sound that begins "like," "Lee," and "low." [l] is also a buzzing sound (voiced), a tongue tip sound (alveolar), and a flowing sound (liquid and glides).

TOUCH CUE: Lay the client's fingertip on the middle of his or her top lip.

DEMONSTRATIONS:

Place (Alveolar)

First Method: Ask the client to feel the bump on the roof of his or her mouth just behind the two front teeth.

Second Method: Place a little peanut butter or a favored food on a Q-tip, touch the Q-tip to the alveolar ridge, and ask the client to remove the food with the tongue tip.

Manner (Approximant)

First Method: Use a strip of paper, a feather, or the hand held in front of the client's mouth while you produce several glides or liquids to draw attention to the "flowing" quality and continuous nature of the sounds. Alternately, tape a small paper flower on the end of a pencil and encourage the client to move the flower in the wind.

Second Method: Run your or the client's finger down the client's arm while making several long glides or liquids to demonstrate the "flowing" quality and length of this sound.

Air Flow (Lateral)

First Method: Place a straw on the groove of the tongue and blow out to demonstrate central emission of air. Place one straw at each corner of the mouth to demonstrate lateral emission of air.

Second Method: Ask the client to breathe in with the tongue as for [s]. Cool air is felt at the central groove. Alternately, perform the straw technique above, remove the straw, and ask the client to breathe in. For lateral sounds, ask the client to breathe in with the tongue in position for [l]. Cool air should be felt on the sides of the tongue over which the air was emitted. An alternate method is to perform the straw technique above, remove the straws, and ask the client to breathe in.

[ɚ]

DESCRIPTION: For retroflex [ɚ], draw attention to the tongue tip raised and curled slightly back and the slight raising of the tongue toward the roof of the mouth. For humped [ɚ], draw attention to the tongue tip being down and the sides of the tongue touching the insides of the back teeth.

Two Types of [r] and [ɚ]

[r] and [ɚ] can be produced in two-ways — retroflex or humped. Some clinicians prefer to facilitate retroflex [ɚ] and [r], others prefer humped [ɚ] and [r].

METAPHORS: The mad dog sound (grrr), the growling tiger sound (grr), or the arm wrestling sound (errr). The sound that ends "hear," "purr," and "car." [ɚ] is also a buzzing sound (voiced) and a tongue tip sound.

TOUCH CUE. None. [ɚ] is usually acquired too late in development for touch cue techniques to be appropriate.

DEMONSTRATIONS:

Same as for [r].

[r]

DESCRIPTION: For retroflex [r], draw attention to the tongue tip curled slightly back and raised toward the bump behind the front teeth. The sides of the tongue are against the sides of the teeth, and the voice box is buzzing. For humped [r], draw attention to the tongue tip being down, the back of the tongue humped up (arched) toward the soft palate, the sides of the tongue lying against the sides of the teeth, and the voice box buzzing.

METAPHORS: The starting race car sound (ruh) and the sound that begins "run," "read," and "red." [r] is also a buzzing sound (voiced), a tongue tip sound (alveolar), and a flowing sound (liquid).

TOUCH CUE: None. [r] is usually acquired too late in development for the touch cue techniques to be appropriate.

DEMONSTRATIONS:

Place (Alveolar)

First Method: Have the client cup his or her hand to indicate that the tongue tip is raised and slightly curled back.

Second Method: Ask the client to feel the bump on the roof of his or her mouth just behind the two front teeth.

Third Method: Place a little peanut butter or a favored food on a Q-tip, touch the Q-tip to the alveolar ridge, and ask the client to remove the food with the tongue tip.

Manner (Approximant)

First Method: Use a strip of paper, a feather, or the hand held in front of the client's mouth while you produce several glides or liquids to draw attention to the "flowing" quality and continuous nature of the sound. Alternately, tape a small paper flower on the end of a pencil and encourage the client to move the flower in the wind.

Second Method: Run your or the client's finger down the client's arm while making several long glides or liquids to demonstrate the "flowing" quality and length of this sound.

[tʃ] and [dʒ]

DESCRIPTION: Draw attention to the contact between the tongue blade and roof of the mouth just behind the bumpy ridge behind the upper front teeth and the way the sound ends in [ʃ]. Additionally, the voice is on for [dʒ], and the sound ends in [ʒ].

METAPHORS: [tʃ] is the choo-choo sound or the sneezing sound (choo!) and the sound that begins "choo-choo train," "chocolate chips," and "cheese." [dʒ] is the motor boat sound and the sound that begins "jump," "joke," and "Joe." Both sounds are back-of-the-hill sounds (postalveolar) and engine chugging sounds (affricate). [dʒ] is made with the voice on (voiced).

DEMONSTRATIONS:

Place (Postalveolar)

First Method: Ask the client to run his or her tongue to where the bump on the roof of the mouth just begins to go down toward the back of the mouth (an analogy of a "hill and valley" can be used).

Second Method: Place a little peanut butter or a favored food on a Q-tip, touch the Q-tip to the postalveolar region, and ask the client to remove the food with his or her tongue blade.

Manner (Affricate)

First Method: Have the client hold his or her hands together tightly and then separate them quickly to indicate the stop onset and fricative release of affricates.

Second Method: Hold the client's hands together and then release them suddenly to indicate the stop onset and fricative release of affricates.

[ʃ] and [ʒ]

DESCRIPTION: Draw attention to the friction noise and the place where the tongue blade touches the roof of the mouth just behind the bumpy ridge behind the upper front teeth. For [ʒ], the voice is on.

METAPHORS: The hushing sound (shh!) or the quiet sound, and the sound that begins "shoe," "sheep," and "show." [ʒ] is the motor sound (zzzz) and the sound in "measure," "beige," and "pleasure." Both [ʃ] and [ʒ] are also back-of-the-hill sounds (postalveolar) and long sounds (fricative). The voice is on (voiced) for [ʒ].

TOUCH CUE: Lay the client's finger in front of his or her lips.

DEMONSTRATIONS:

Place (Postalveolar)

First Method: Ask the client to run the tongue to where the bump on the mouth roof just begins to go down toward the back of the mouth (an analogy of a "hill and valley" can be used).

Second Method: Place a little peanut butter or a favored food on a Q-tip, touch the Q-tip to the postalveolar region, and ask the client to remove the food with the tongue blade.

Manner (Fricative)

First Method: Use a strip of paper, a feather, or the hand held in front of the client's mouth while you produce several long voiceless fricatives to draw attention to the "hissing" quality and continuous nature of the sounds. Alternately, tape a small paper flower on the end of a pencil and encourage the client to move the flower in the wind.

Second Method: Run your or the client's finger down the client's arm while making several long voiceless fricatives to demonstrate the "hissing" quality and length of fricatives.

[j]

DESCRIPTION: Draw attention to the flowing air and the slight rise of the middle of the tongue toward the roof of the mouth. The voice is on.

METAPHORS: The "yes" sound and the sound that begins "yes," "you," and "year." [j] is also a flowing sound (glides and liquids), a middle sound (palatal), and the voice is on (voiced).

TOUCH CUES: None.

DEMONSTRATIONS:

Place (Palatal)

First Method: Ask the client to run his or her tongue backward from the bump to the highest point on the roof of the mouth.

Second Method: Place a little peanut butter or a favored food on a Q-tip, and touch the Q-tip to the arch of the hard palate. Ask the client to remove the food with his or her tongue blade.

Third Method: Touch the middle of the tongue lightly with a tongue depressor and ask the client to hump up that part of the tongue toward the roof of the mouth.

Manner (Approximant)

First Method: Use a strip of paper, a feather, or the hand held in front of the client's mouth while you produce several glides or liquids to draw attention to the "flowing" quality and continuous nature of the sounds. Alternately, tape a small paper flower on the end of a pencil and encourage the client to move the flower in the wind.

Second Method: Run your or the client's finger down the client's arm while making several long glides or liquids to demonstrate the "flowing" quality and length of this sound.

[k] and [g]

DESCRIPTION: Draw attention to the back of the tongue touching the back of the roof of the mouth, the quick separation of the articulators, and the air flowing out the mouth. [k] is made with the voice off, and [g] is made with the voice on.

METAPHORS: [k] is the coughing sound and the sound that begins "cold," "king," and "kite." [g] is the water pouring sound (glug, glug, glug) or the "greaat!" (Tony the Tiger) sound, and the sound that begins "go," "goat," and "gate." Both [k] and [g] are also quick sounds (stops) and tongue-back sounds (velar). [k] is a voice-off sound (voiceless), and [g] is a voice-on sound (voiced).

TOUCH CUE: Lay the client's finger at the uppermost part of his or her neck.

DEMONSTRATIONS:

Place (Velar)

First Method: Place the client's hand in contact with the underside of your mouth and repeat [k] several times while drawing attention to the muscle movements.

Second Method: Open your mouth and allow the client to observe while you say [k] several times.

Manner (Oral Stop)

First Method: Use a strip of paper, a feather, or the hand held in front of the client's mouth while you produce a series of stops to demonstrate the explosive release of stops. Alternately, tape a small paper flower on the end a pencil and encourage the client to move the flower with puffs of air.

Second Method: Place your or the client's palms together and then suddenly separate them to demonstrate the sudden release of stops.

[ŋ]

DESCRIPTION: Draw attention to the back of the tongue touching the back of the roof of the mouth, the air flowing through the nose, and the voice being on.

METAPHORS: The gong sound and the sound that ends "sing," "wing," and "ring." [ŋ] is also a back tongue sound (velar), a voice-on sound (voiced), and a nose sound (nasal).

TOUCH CUE: Lay the client's finger at uppermost part of his or her neck.

DEMONSTRATIONS:

Place (Velar)

First Method: Place the client's hand in contact with the underside of your mouth and repeat [ŋ] several times while drawing attention to the muscle movements.

Second Method: Open your mouth and allow the client to observe while you say [ŋ] several times.

Manner (Nasal Stop)

First Method: Contrast breathing through the nose onto a mirror or a piece of paper with breathing through the mouth onto a mirror or piece of paper.

Second Method: Instruct the client to take a deep breath, hold it, and let air out through the nose to produce a voiceless nasal sound.

Third Method: To demonstrate nasality with voicing, instruct the client to take a deep breath, hold it, and say "ah" with the mouth closed so that air comes out the nose. Telling the client to open his or her mouth will help teach release of a nasal consonant.

[h]

DESCRIPTION: Draw attention to the hissing sound in the throat.

METAPHORS: The panting dog sound and the sound that begins "hug," "happy," and "ho" (Santa Claus' ho-ho-ho). [h] is also a long sound (fricative) and a voice-off sound (voiceless).

TOUCH CUES: None.

DEMONSTRATIONS:

Place (Glottal)

First Method: Point to your larynx while making [h] or a vowel.

Second Method: Instruct the client to touch his or her larynx between the first finger and thumb and swallow.

Manner (Approximant)

First Method. Use a strip of paper, a feather, or the hand held in front of the client's mouth while you produce several glides or liquids to draw attention to the "flowing" quality and continuous nature of the sound. Alternately, tape a small paper flower on the end of a pencil and encourage the client to move the flower in the wind.

Second Method: Run your or the client's finger down the client's arm while making several long glides or liquids to demonstrate the "flowing" quality and length of this sound.

Appendix 5B

Word Pairs[1]

A. Introduction

This appendix is designed to use in contrast therapy activities like those described earlier in this chapter. A chart showing the feature differences between treatment target sounds and other possible sounds begins on the following page. The feature differences are those of place, manner, and voicing (Williams, 1993). The remainder of the appendix consists of four lists of word pairs showing:

Word pairs for word-initial consonants,

Word pairs for cluster deletion and cluster reduction in word-initial position,

Word pairs for cluster reduction in word-final position, and

Word pairs for consonant substitutions in word-final position.

The words in the lists that follow are common nouns, common verbs, letters of the alphabet, and names from popular storybooks. For certain sounds, no words were found that met the above criteria, and the list was left blank. Extra spaces are provided at the end of each list for clinicians to add their own preferred words.

---

[1]This appendix is adapted from S. Walsh (Walsh, 1994).

B. Chart of Feature Differences

Sound	One Feature	Two Features	Three Features
p	b t k	d g f θ s ʃ tʃ m w h	v ð z ʒ dʒ n ŋ l r j
b	p d g m w	t k v ð z ʒ dʒ n ŋ l r j	f θ s ʃ tʃ h
t	p d k s	b g f θ z ʃ tʃ n l r h	v ð ʒ dʒ m ŋ j w
d	b t g z n l r	p k v ð s ʒ dʒ m ŋ j w	f θ ʃ tʃ h
k	p t g	b d f θ s ʃ tʃ ŋ h	v ð z ʒ dʒ m n l r j w
g	b d k ŋ	p t v ð z ʒ dʒ m n l r j w	f θ s ʃ tʃ h
f	v θ s ʃ	p t k ð z ʒ tʃ h	b d g dʒ m n ŋ l r j w
v	f ð z ʒ	b d g θ s ʃ dʒ m n ŋ l r j w	p t k tʃ h
θ	f ð s ʃ	p t k v z ʒ tʃ h	b d g dʒ m n ŋ l r j w
ð	v θ z ʒ	b d g f s ʃ dʒ m n ŋ l r j w	p t k tʃ h
s	f θ z ʃ t	p d k v ð ʒ tʃ n l r h	b g dʒ m ŋ j w
z	d v ð s ʒ n l r	b t g f θ ʃ dʒ m j w ŋ	p k tʃ h
ʃ	f θ s ʒ tʃ	p t k v ð z dʒ h	b d g m n ŋ l r j w
ʒ	v ð z ʃ dʒ	b d g f θ s tʃ m n ŋ l r j w	p t k h

continued

Chart of Feature Differences *(continued)*

Sound	One Feature	Two Features	Three Features
tʃ	ʃ dʒ	p t k f θ s ʒ h	b d g v ð z m n ŋ l r j w
dʒ	ʒ tʃ	b d g v ð z ʃ m n ŋ l r j w	p t k f θ s h
m	n ŋ b w	p d g v ð z ʒ dʒ l r j	t k f θ s ʃ tʃ h
n	d z m ŋ l r	b t g v ð s ʒ dʒ j w	p k f ʃ tʃ h θ
ŋ	m n g	b d k v ð z ʒ dʒ l r j w	p t f θ s ʃ tʃ h
l	d z n r	b t g v ð s ʒ dʒ m ŋ j w	p k f θ ʃ tʃ h
r	d n z l	b t g v ð s ʒ dʒ m ŋ j w	p k f θ ʃ tʃ h
j	w	b d g v ð z ʒ dʒ m n ŋ l r h	p t k f θ ɛ ʃ tʃ
w	b m j	p d g v ð z ʒ dʒ n ŋ l r h	t k f θ s ʃ tʃ
h		p t k f θ s ʃ tʃ j w	b d g v ð z ʒ dʒ m n ŋ l r

C. Word-Initial Contrasts

[p]

Sound	1 Feature	2 Features	3 Features
pear	bear, tear	hair, wear	
pea	key, bee	sea	knee, z
peas	keys	cheese	knees
potato	tomato		
pie	bye, tie	high, thigh	
peach	beach, teach		reach
pig	big	wig, dig	
pan	can	fan, man	ran
pin		fin, chin, thin, win	
parrot	carrot		
pat	cat, bat	mat, sat, hat, fat	rat
pen	ten	men, hen	
pet		wet	vet, net, jet
pond		wand	
pay		day, hay, weigh	ray, neigh
pickle	tickle		nickel
*pog		dog	log
paste	taste	waist, chased	raced
poke		soak, choke	joke, yolk
pail	tail	sail, mail, whale	nail, jail, rail, veil
purse			nurse
pick	tick, kick	sick, wick, thick	lick
paw			jaw
pink		sink, wink, think	rink
pull	bull	wool	
pop	top, cop	mop, hop, chop, shop	

continued

[p] *(continued)*

Sound	1 Feature	2 Features	3 Features
pearl		girl	
pave	cave	wave, shave	
pot		hot, dot	
peel		deal, meal, seal, wheel	
path	bath	math	
pest	test	chest, west	vest, nest
pour	core	four, door	roar
park	bark	shark, dark	
post	toast	ghost	roast
pill	bill	hill	
peep	keep, beep	deep, sheep, cheap	jeep, leap
pool	tool, cool	fool	jewel
——	——	——	——
——	——	——	——

¹ pog: A pog is a term used to refer to milk caps, which are used to play a game in Hawaii and often are given to children as reinforcement in place of stickers.

[b]

Sound	1 Feature	2 Features	3 Features
bee	pea	knee, z, key	sea
bug	mug	rug, jug	hug
bear	pear		hair
bird	word	nerd	third, heard
bunny	money		funny, honey, sunny
bat	mat, pat	cat, rat	fat, hat, sat
bye	pie	tie	high, thigh, sigh
big	dig, pig, wig		
box		rocks	fox, socks
bed	dead	red	head
beach	peach	reach, teach	
bow	go, mow	toe, row, no	sew, hoe
bows		toes, rose, nose	hose
boat	goat	coat, note	
ball	wall	call, tall	hall, fall
bone		cone	phone
boy		toy	
bad	mad, dad		sad
bake		cake, lake	
boo	goo, moo	two, zoo, new	shoe, chew
beef		leaf	thief, chief
book		cook, look	hook
bump		jump	hump
bath	path, math		
bell			shell
belt	melt		
bite	white	night, light, kite, write	fight

continued

[b] *(continued)*

Sound	1 Feature	2 Features	3 Features
bark	park, dark		shark
bill	pill		hill
beans		jeans	
berry			cherry, hairy, fairy
bull	wool, pull		
band		tanned	hand, sand, fanned
boom		zoom, room	
beep	deep, peep	leap, jeep, keep	sheep, cheep
bun	one	run	fun, sun

[t]

Sound	1 Feature	2 Features	3 Features
tomato	potato		
ten	pen	hen	men
tickle	pickle	nickel	
toast	post	ghost, roast	
taste	paste	chased, raced	waist
tail	pail, sail	nail, rail	mail, whale, jail, veil
teach	peach	reach, beach	
toes		rose, nose, hose, bows	
tear	pear	hair, bear	
tie	pie	high, bye, thigh	
tick	kick, pick, sick	thick, lick	wick
talk		chalk, hawk	walk
top	pop, cop	hop, chop, shop	mop
tool	cool, pool	fool	jewel
tall	call	ball, fall, hall	wall
time	dime		
toy		boy	
two		chew, goo, boo, new, zoo, shoe	moo
tire		fire	
tube	cube		
tear	deer	cheer, fear, hear	year
tanned	sand	hand, band, fanned	
test		nest, chest	west, vest
toe	sew	bow, row, go hoe, no	mow

[d]

Sound	1 Feature	2 Features	3 Features
dog	log	pog[a]	
dig	big	wig, pig	
dish		wish	fish
dime	time		
dad	bad	mad, sad	
dot		pot	hot
dart		cart	heart
dive			hive, five
door	roar	core, pour	four
dark	bark	park	shark
deal		peel, meal, wheel, seal	
day	neigh, ray	pay, weigh	hay
dawn	lawn	yawn	fawn
deer	tear	year, peer	hear, fear, cheer
dirt			shirt, hurt
deep	beep, leap	peep, keep, jeep	sheep, cheep, heap
dead	bed, red		head
dust	rust		

---

[a] pog: A pog is a term used to refer to milk caps, which are used to play a game in Hawaii and often are given to children as reinforcement in place of stickers.

[k]

Sound	1 Feature	2 Features	3 Features
can	pan	fan	man
carrot	parrot		
keys	peas	cheese	knees
king		sing	ring, wing
kick	tick, pick	sick, thick	wick, lick
cop	pop, top	shop, hop, chop	mop
cat	pat	bat, sat, hat, fat	rat, mat
cool	pool, tool	fool	jewel
cut			nut
coat	goat	boat	note
call	tall	fall, hall, ball	wall
key	pea	bee, sea	knee
cone		phone, bone	
cake		bake	lake
cold	gold	hold, fold	mold, rolled
cave	pave	shave	wave
cart		dart, heart	
cook		book, hook	look
camp		lamp	
kite		bite, fight	write, white, light, night
candle		handle, sandal	
cube	tube		
curled			world
corn	torn	thorn, horn	worn
core	pour	door, four	roar
card	guard	hard	yard
keep	peep	deep, beep, cheep, sheep	jeep, leap
calf		half	laugh

[g]

Sound	1 Feature	2 Features	3 Features
goat	boat, coat	note	
girl		pearl	
gold	cold	mold, rolled	fold, hold
goo	boo	two, zoo, new, moo	chew, shoe
ghost		toast, post, roast	
gum			thumb
gasoline		Vaseline	
guard	card	yard	hard
go	bow	toe, row, mow, no	sew, hoe
gun	bun	run, one	sun, fun
————	————	————	————
————	————	————	————

[f]

Sound	1 Feature	2 Features	3 Features
fan		pan, can	man
fin	thin	pin, chin	win
fat	sat	cat, pat, hat	bat, mat, rat
fox	socks		box, rocks
fish			dish, wish
fun	sun		run, one, gun
feather			leather
fool		tool, pool, cool	jewel
fall		tall, call, hall	ball, wall
phone		cone	bone
fold		cold, hold	mold, rolled, gold
five		hive	dive
funny	sunny	honey	money, bunny
fell	shell		bell
four		core, pour	door, roar
fight		kite	white, night, write, bite, light
fire		tire	
fourth			north
fawn			lawn, yawn, dawn
fear		tear, cheer, hear	near, deer
fanned	sand	tanned, hand	band
fairy		cherry, hairy	berry
face		chase	race, lace

[v]

Sound	1 Feature	2 Features	3 Features
vest		nest, west	test, chest, pest
vine		shine, nine, sign, line	
Vaseline		gasoline	
veil		rail, mail, sail, whale, nail	pail, hail, tail
vet		wet, net, jet	pet
vein		mane, rain	
_____	_____	_____	_____
_____	_____	_____	_____

[θ]

Sound	1 Feature	2 Features	3 Features
thin		chin, pin	
thick	sick	pick, tick, kick	wick, lick
think	sink	pink	wink, rink
thief		chief	beef, leaf
thumb			gum
thigh		tie, pie, high	bye
thunder			wonder
thorn		corn, torn, horn	worn
thong	song		long
third		heard	word, bird, nerd
_____	_____	_____	_____
_____	_____	_____	_____

[ð]

Sound	1 Feature	2 Features	3 Features
No words selected			

[s]

Sound	1 Feature	2 Features	3 Features
sat	fat	pat, rat, cat, hat	mat, bat
sail	tail	pail, nail, veil, rail	whale, mail, jail
socks	fox	rocks	box
soap		rope	
sew	toe	row, hoe, no	bow, mow, go
sun	fun	run	one, bun, gun
sick	tick, thick	kick, pick, lick	wick
sink	think	pink, rink	wink
sea		pea, knee, key	bee
sad		dad	bad, mad
six		chicks	mix
seal		peel, deal	wheel, meal
sunny	funny	honey	money, bunny
sand	fanned, tanned	hand	band
Sam[a]		ham, lamb	jam
sign	shine	vine, nine, line	
sandal		handle, candle	
song	thong	long	
soak		poke, choke	yolk, joke, woke
sew	toe	row	go, bow
sing		king, ring	wing
sip	zip, ship	lip, hip, dip, rip	whip

[a] Sam: Sam is a character in the Dr. Seuss book, *Green Eggs and Ham.*

[z]

Sound	1 Feature	2 Features	3 Features
zoo	new	shoe, two, moo, goo, boo	chew
zip	lip, sip, rip	whip, ship	chip, hip
zero			hero
zoom	room	boom	
z	knee, sea	bee	pea, key

[ʃ]

Sound	1 Feature	2 Features	3 Features
shirt		hurt	dirt
shoe	chew	zoo, two	goo, boo, moo, new
ship	chip, sip	hip, zip	whip, rip, lip
shark		park	bark, dark
shine	sign	vine	nine, line
shell	fell		bell
shop	chop	pop, top, cop, hop	mop
shave		pave, cave	wave
sheep	cheep	keep, peep, jeep	deep, leap

[tʃ]

Sound	1 Feature	2 Features	3 Features
chased		paste, taste	raced, waist
chase		face	race, lace
chin		pin, thin	
cheese		peas, keys	knees
chip	ship	hip, sip	rip, lip, whip, zip, dip
chunk	junk		
chop	shop	cop, pop, top, hop	mop
chew	shoe	two	moo, goo, boo, zoo
chief		thief	beef, leaf
chicks		six	mix
chest		pest, test	vest, nest, west
cherry		fairy, hairy	berry
chalk		talk, hawk	walk
cheer		fear, hear, tear	deer, year, near
cheep	sheep, jeep		deep, leap
choke	joke	soak, poke	yolk

[dʒ]

Sound	1 Feature	2 Features	3 Features
jug		bug, mug	
jail		nail, whale, mail	pail, sail, tail
jaw			paw
junk	chunk		
jewel			fool, cool, tool, pool
Jello		yellow	
jacket		racket	
jump		bump	hump
jam		lamb	ham, Sam[a]
jeans		beans	
jeep	cheep	deep, sheep, leap, beep	keep, peep
germ		worm	
gym		limb	him
jel		wel, nel, vel	pel
joke	choke	yolk	poke, soak
————	————	————	————
————	————	————	————

[a] Sam: Sam is a character in the Dr. Seuss book, *Green Eggs and Ham.*

[m]

Sound	1 Feature	2 Features	3 Features
man		pan	fan, can
mat	bat	pat, rat	fat, hat, cat, sat
mug	bug	jug, rug	hug
mail	whale, nail	pail, jail, rail, veil	sail, tail
men		pen	hen, ten
mouse			house
mice		rice	
mop		pop	shop, chop, top, cop, hop
mad	bad	dad	sad
mold		gold, rolled	hold, fold, cold
moo	new, boo	goo, zoo	chew, two, shoe
meal	wheel	peel, deal	seal
money	bunny		funny, honey, sunny
math	bath	path	
melt	belt		
mow	no	go, row	toe, hoe, sew
mix			six, chicks
mane		rain, vein	

[n]

Sound	1 Feature	2 Features	3 Features
nail	mail, rail	jail, whale, veil, sail, tail	pail
knees		peas, cheese, keys	
nose	rose	toes, bows	hose
nurse			purse
knock	rock, lock	sock	
nut			cut
note		boat, goat	coat
knee	z	sea (see), bee	pea, key
nest		vest, west, test	pest, chest
night	write, light	white, bite	fight, kite
nine	line	vine, sign	shine
neigh	day, ray	weigh	hay, pay
north			fourth
net		vet, wet, jet	pet
near	deer	year, tear	hear, fear, cheer
no	mow, row	go, sew, toe, bow	hoe
nerd		word, bird	third, heard
nickel		tickle	pickle

[l]

Sound	1 Feature	2 Features	3 Features
log	dog		pog[a]
leather			feather
lick		sick, tick, wick	pick, kick, thick
lock	rock, knock	sock	
lake		bake	cake
look		book	cook, hook
lip	zip, rip, dip	whip, sip	chip, ship, hip
lamp			camp
light	night, write	white, bite	fight, kite
line	nine	vine, sign	shine
long		song	thong
late		wait	
lawn	dawn	yawn	
leap	deep	jeep	heap, cheep, sheep, keep, peep
laugh			calf, half
limb		gym	him
life	knife	wife	
leaf			chief, thief
lamb		jam, Sam[b]	ham
lace	race		chase, face

[a] pog: A pog is a term used to refer to milk caps, which are used to play a game in Hawaii and often are given to children as reinforcement in place of stickers.

[b] Sam: Sam is a character in the Dr. Seuss book, *Green Eggs and Ham*.

[r]

Sound	1 Feature	2 Features	3 Features
rat		sat, mat, bat	pat, fat, hat, cat
rug		mug, bug, jug	hug
roast		toast	
raced		taste	chased, paste
rocks		socks, box	fox
red	dead	bed	head
reach		beach, teach	
rose	nose	toes, bows	
ring		sing, wing	king
rice		mice	
rope		soap	
row	no	bow, toe, mow, go, sew	
run		sun, bun, one, gun	fun
rink		sink, wink	think, pink
rock	lock, knock	sock	
rug		mug, bug	hug
rolled		mold, gold	fold, hold, cold
roar	door		core, four, pour
rip	zip, lip, dip	whip, sip	ship, chip, hip
racket		jacket	
write	night, light	bite, white	fight, kite
rain		vein, mane	
rust	dust		
race	lace		chase, face
room	zoom	boom	
rail	nail	whale, mail, sail, jail, veil, tail	pail
ray	day, neigh	weigh	pay, hay
___	___	___	___
___	___	___	___

[j]

Sound	1 Feature	2 Features	3 Features
yellow		Jello	
yard		guard, hard	card
yolk	woke	joke	poke, soak, choke
yawn		dawn, lawn	fawn
year		deer, hear	tear, fear, cheer
————	————	————	————
————	————	————	————

[w]

Sound	1 Feature	2 Features	3 Features
whale	mail	nail, pail, jail, rail, veil	sail, tail
wing		ring	king
one	bun	run, gun	fun, sun
wand		pond	
wick		pick, lick	kick, tick, sick, thick
wish		dish	fish
wink		pink, rink	think, sink
walk		hawk	chalk, talk
wall	ball	hall	fall, tall, call
wave		pave	shave, cave
wheel	meal	peel, heel	seal
whip		zip, rip, dip, lip, hip	chip, sip, ship
white	bite	write, night, light	fight, kite
world			curled
wonder			thunder
wet		net, vet, pet, jet	
wool	bull	pull	
worm		germ	
wand		pond	
wife		knife, life	
word	bird	nerd, heard	third
west		pest, nest, vest	chest, test
waist		raced, paced	taste, chased
wig	big	pig, dig	
weigh		ray, day, pay, neigh, hay	
wait		late	

[h]

Sound	1 Feature	2 Features	3 Features
hat		pat, cat, fat, sat	bat, rat, mat
hair		pear, wear	bear
hurt		shirt	
hen		pen, ten	men
house			mouse
hair		tear	
head			bed, dead, red
hand		tanned, sand, fanned	band
hawk		chalk, talk, walk	
hop		top, cop, chop, pop, shop	mop
hall		tall, fall, wall	mall
heard		third, word	nerd, bird
hug		tug	bug, mug, rug, jug
hold		cold, fold	mold, rolled, gold
hot		pot	dot
heart		cart	dart
hive		five	dive
honey		sunny, funny	bunny, money
hook		cook	book, look
him			gym, limb
hip		chip, ship, sip, whip	rip, lip, zip
hump			bump, jump, lump
ham			jam, lamb
hill		pill	bill
handle		candle, sandal	
hay		pay, weigh	day, neigh, lay, ray
high		thigh	

continued

[h] *(continued)*

Sound	1 Feature	2 Features	3 Features
hairy		cherry, fairy	berry
horn		corn, thorn	
hard		card, yard	guard
hear		cheer, peer, fear	year, deer
hero			zero
hurt		shirt	dirt
half		calf	laugh
head			dead, red
hoe		sew, toe	row, go, mow, no
hose		toes	rose, nose, bows
_____	_____	_____	_____
_____	_____	_____	_____

D. Cluster Reduction

[l] Clusters

Sound	Word	1st Consonant	2nd or 3rd Consonant
[pl]	plane	pain	
	plants	pants	
	play	pay	lay
	please	peas	
	plate		late
	_____	_____	_____
	_____	_____	_____
[kl]	clip		lip
	club	cub	
	clock		lock
	clap	cap	lap
	cluck		luck
	cloud		loud
	clam		lamb
	claw	caw	
	climb		lime
	_____	_____	_____
	_____	_____	_____
[bl]	black	back	
	blue	boo	
	bleed	bead	lead
	block		lock
	blank	bank	
	_____	_____	_____
	_____	_____	_____

continued

[l] Clusters *(continued)*

Sound	Word	1st Consonant	2nd or 3rd Consonant
[gl]	glass	gas	
	glitter		litter
	globe		lobe (ear)
	glow		low
	glue	goo	
[fl]	floor	four	
	flight	fight	light
	flat	fat	
	flash		lash (eye)
	flip		lip
[sl]	slip	sip	lip
	slide	side	
	sleep		leap
	sleeve		leave
	sliver		liver

[r] Clusters

Sound	Word	1st Consonant	2nd or 3rd Consonant
[pr]	prize	pies	rise
	price		rice
	prince		rinse
	pray		ray
	prick	pick	
[tr]	trip		rip
	track	tack	rack
	train		rain
	tree	tea	
	tray		ray
	trap	tap	rap
	trail	tail	rail
	trash		rash
	trick	tick	
	troll		roll
[kr]	crab	cab	
	crib		rib
	crow		row
	crash	cash	rash
	croak	Coke (soda)	
	crust		rust

continued

[r] Clusters *(continued)*

Sound	Word	1st Consonant	2nd or 3rd Consonant
[br]	bread	bed	red
	broom	boom	room
	branch		ranch
	brake	bake	rake
	brain		rain
[dr]	drink		rink
	drive	dive	
	driver	diver	
	drill	dill	
	drawer	door	roar
	drag		rag
	drip	dip	rip
[gr]	grass	gas	
	grease	geese	
	great	gate	
	ground		round
	gray		ray
	grow	go	row
[fr]	front		runt
	fruit		root
	frog	fog	
[θr]	three	tree	
	throw		row
	thread		red

[w] Clusters

Sound	Word	1st Consontant	2nd or 3rd Consonant
[tw]	twig		wig
	twin	tin	win
	_____	_____	_____
	_____	_____	_____
[kw]	quick	kick	wick
	quack		whack
	quake	cake	wake
	_____	_____	_____
	_____	_____	_____
[sw]	see **[s] Clusters**		

[s] Clusters

Sound	Word	1st Consonant	2nd or 3rd Consonant
[sp]	spot		pot
	spout		pout
	spool		pool
	spill		pill
	spit	sit	pit
	spark		park
	spin		pin
	spade		paid
	spy		pie
	_____	_____	_____
	_____	_____	_____
[st]	stop		top
	sting	sing	
	stink	sink	
	stack	sack	tack
	stick	sick	tick
	stair		tear
	steam		team
	stool		tool
	steal	seal	
	stale	sail	tail
	stand	sand	
	stub	sub	tub
	star		tar
	stew		two
	_____	_____	_____
	_____	_____	_____

Sound	Word	1st Consonant	2nd or 3rd Consonant
[sk]	school		cool
	ski	sea	key
	scale	sail	
	skunk	sunk	
	skip	sip	
[sw]	swing	sing	wing
	sweat	set	wet
	sweet	seat	
	switch		witch
[sm]	small		mall
	smell	sell	
	smile		mile
	smoke	soak	
	smack	sack	
[sn]	snack	sack	
	snail	sail	nail
	snow	sew	no
	snap		nap
	sneeze		knees
[sl]	see [l] Clusters		

continued

[s] Clusters *(continued)*

Sound	Word	1st Consonant	2nd or 3rd Consonant
[spr]	spring	sing	ring
	spray		ray, pay, pray
	Sprite (soda)		write, white
	sprinkle		wrinkle
[str]	struck	suck	truck
	strong	song	wrong
	street	seat	treat
	string	sting, sing	
	stream	steam	team
	strap		trap, rap (music)
[skr]	scream		cream
[skw]	square		wear
	squash		wash
	squeal	seal	wheel
	squeak		weak
[spl]	No words selected		

[ʃr]

Sound	Word	1st Consonant	2nd or 3rd Consonant
[ʃr]	shrub		rub
	shred		red
	shrug		rug
	_____	_____	_____
	_____	_____	_____

E. Final Consonant Deletion

Oral Stops

Sound	Word	Deletion
[p]	rope	row
	keep	key
	sheep	she
	soap	sew
	type	tie
	peep	pea
	pipe	pie
	_____	_____
	_____	_____
[b]	robe	row
	tube	two
	cob	caw
	rob	raw
	_____	_____
	_____	_____
[t]	goat	go
	date	day
	boat	bow
	beet	bee
	shoot	shoe
	seat	sea
	note	no
	plate	play
	toot	two
	boot	boo
	ate	A
	moat	mow
	bite	buy
	_____	_____
	_____	_____

Sound	Word	Deletion
[d]	road	row
	toad	toe
	seed	sea
	bead	bee
	dude	do
	_____	_____
	_____	_____
[k]	cake	K
	peek	pea
	rake	ray
	bike	buy
	beak	B
	back	baa
	_____	_____
	_____	_____
[g]	jog	jaw
	pog	paw
	egg	A
	_____	_____
	_____	_____

Fricatives

Sound	Word	Deletion
[f]	goof	goo
	roof	Roo (Winnie the Poo)
	leaf	Ali (Alladin)
[v]	move	moo
	dive	die
	wave	weigh
	cave	K
[θ]	bath	baa
	teeth	tea
	tooth	two
[ð]	No words selected	
[s]	dice	die
	moose	moo
	ice	eye
	race	ray
	gross	grow

Sound	Word	Deletion
[z]	nose	no
	rose	row
	hose	hoe
	toes	toe
	shoes	shoe
	maze	May
	crows	crow
	bows	bow
	_____	_____
	_____	_____
[ʃ]	No words selected	
	_____	_____
[ʒ]	No words selected	
	_____	_____

Affricates

Sound	Word	Deletion
[tʃ]	teach	tea
	peach	pea
	beach	bee
	couch	cow
	___	___
	___	___
[dʒ]	cage	K
	page	pay
	badge	baa
	___	___
	___	___

Nasal Stops

Sound	Word	Deletion
[m]	boom	boo
	time	tie
	dime	die
	home	hoe
	broom	brew
	zoom	zoo
[n]	moon	moo
	bone	bow
	cane	K
	rain	ray
	bean	bee (B)
[ŋ]	song	saw
	thong	thaw
	sing	sea
	king	key

Liquids

Sound	Word	Deletion
[l]	roll	row
	bowl	bow
	rail	ray
	tile	tie
	dial	die
	seal	sea
	hole	hoe
	pile	pie
	mole	mow
	peel	P
	cool	coo
	nail	neigh
	pail	pay
	goal	go

F. Final Consonant Substitutions

[p]

Sound	1 Feature	2 Features	3 Features
cap	cab, cat	catch, calf	can
map	mat	match, math, mad, mash	man
cup	cut		
hop	hot	hog	
rope		road	rose, roll
beep	beet, beak	beach, bead, beef	bees, bean
lip	lick		
leap	leak	leave, leaf, leash, leech	lean
_____	_____	_____	_____
_____	_____	_____	_____

[b]

Sound	1 Feature	2 Features	3 Features
cab	cap	cat, can	catch, calf
web		wet	
_____	_____	_____	_____
_____	_____	_____	_____

continued

[t]

Sound	1 Feature	2 Features	3 Features
cut	cup		
hot	hop	hog	
cat	cap	catch, can, cab, calf	
beet	beep, beak, bead	beach, bean, bees, beef	
boat		bone	
bat	bad, back	bath	badge
mat	mad, map	math, man match	
pat	pack, pass	patch, pan	
tent		tenth	
hat		half, hatch	ham
wet		web	
————	————	————	————
————	————	————	————

[d]

Sound	1 Feature	2 Features	3 Features
bead	bees, bean, beet	beep	beef, beach
road	roll, rose	rope	
toad	toes		
mad	man, mat	map	match, math, mash
bad	bat	back, badge	bath
————	————	————	————
————	————	————	————

[k]

Sound	1 Feature	2 Features	3 Features
hawk			hall
leak	leap	leaf, leech, leash	lean, leave
back	bat	bad, bath	badge
lick	lip		
cheek		chief	cheese
walk		wash, watch	wall
lock	log	long	lawn
rake			rain, rail
sink		sing	
beak	beep, beet	beach, bead, beef	bean, bees
____	____	____	____
____	____	____	____

[g]

Sound	1 Feature	2 Features	3 Features
hog		hot, hop	
log	lock, long	lawn	
____	____	____	____
____	____	____	____

continued

[f]

Sound	1 Feature	2 Features	3 Features
leaf	leave, leash	leap, leak, leech	lean
beef		beep, beak, beach, beet	bean, bead, bees
half		hatch, hat	ham
chief		cheese, cheek	
calf		cat, cap, catch	cab, can
____	____	____	____
____	____	____	____

[v]

Sound	1 Feature	2 Features	3 Features
leave	leaf	leash, lean	leap, leak, leech
____	____	____	____
____	____	____	____

[θ]

Sound	1 Feature	2 Features	3 Features
bath		bat, back	badge, bad
math		mat, map, match	mad, man
tenth		tent	
path	pass	pat, pack, patch	pan
mouth	mouse		
____	____	____	____
____	____	____	____

[ð]

Sound	1 Feature	2 Features	3 Features
	No words selected		

[s]

Sound	1 Feature	2 Features	3 Features
pass	path, pat	pan, pack, patch	
mouse	mouth		

[z]

Sound	1 Feature	2 Features	3 Features
chains		change	
rose	road		rope
bees	bead, bean	beef	beep, beet, beak, beach
toes	toad		
cheese		chief	cheek
bows	bone	boat	

continued

[ʃ]

Sound	1 Feature	2 Features	3 Features
leash	leaf, leech	leap, leak	lead, lean
wash	watch	walk	wall
mash	match		man

[ʒ]

Sound	1 Feature	2 Features	3 Features
	No words selected		

[tʃ]

Sound	1 Feature	2 Features	3 Features
patch		pat, pack, path, pass	pan
match	mash	mat, map, math	man, mad
leech	leash	leak, leaf, leave, leap	lean
beach		beep, beet, beak, beef	bean, bead, bees
hatch		hat, half	ham
watch	wash	walk	wall
catch		calf, cap, cat	can, cab

[dʒ]

Sound	1 Feature	2 Features	3 Features
change		chains	
badge		bad	bat, bath, back
___	___	___	___
___	___	___	___

[m]

Sound	1 Feature	2 Features	3 Features
swim	swing		
ham			half, hat, hatch
gum	gun		
___	___	___	___
___	___	___	___

[n]

Sound	1 Feature	2 Features	3 Features
pan		pat, pass	patch, pack, path
bone	bows	boat	
pin	pill	pit, pig	pick
lawn	long	log	lock
gun	gum		
rain	rail		rake
lean			leash, leap, leak, leaf, leave
can	cab	cat	cap, calf, catch
man	mad	mat	map, match, math, mash
bean	bead, bees	beet	beep, beak, beach, beef
___	___	___	___
___	___	___	___

continued

[ŋ]

Sound	1 Feature	2 Features	3 Features
swing	swim		
long	lawn, log	lock	
sing		sink	
_____	_____	_____	_____
_____	_____	_____	_____

[l]

Sound	1 Feature	2 Features	3 Features
hall			hawk
roll	road, rose		rope
bowl	bone, bows	boat	
wall			wash, watch, walk
rail	rain		rake
tall			talk, top
_____	_____	_____	_____
_____	_____	_____	_____

Appendix 5C

Phonetic Placement and Shaping Techniques

A. Introduction

The following are phonetic placement and shaping techniques for American English consonants and [ɚ]. The instructions are "bare bones" descriptions of techniques that should be studied prior to commencing the treatment session and elaborated on in whatever way seems appropriate to the clinician. An instruction to "touch the client's lips together," for example, might be simply performed or elaborated into a complicated game, depending on the clinician's style and the client's needs.

Shaping techniques that involve common error patterns are indicated by three asterisks (***). For many sounds, more than one technique is described. When this occurs, the methods are listed in approximate order of difficulty, from least to most difficult. When cognates (pairs of sounds differing only in voicing) are presented, the instructions are for the voiceless sound. The voiced sound is facilitated by following the instructions for the voiceless sound and then asking the client to "turn on the voice" or some similar metaphor. The demonstrations of voicing listed in Table 5–5 may also be used to facilitate the production of voicing, for example, with clients with Final Consonant Devoicing, or to facilitate lack of voicing in clients with Prevocalic Voicing.

How to Avoid a Frustrating Situation

The following frustrating situation can arise when performing phonetic placement and shaping techniques. The example describes [t], but the situation can arise with any sound. The clinician carefully and successfully leads the client through all but the last step to produce [t]. Yet, when the clinician says, "Now say [t]," the client moves his or her articulators and reverts to the old pronunciation. Although there is no guaranteed way to keep this situation from arising, the

continued

---

chance of it occurring can be reduced if the clinician uses instructions that do not remind the client of the old pronunciation. After the client's mouth is in position for [t], for example, instead of saying "Now say [t]," the clinician might say, "Now let's play. Lower your tongue quickly" (or some other such instruction). After the client produces the [t]-like sound correctly approximately five times, the clinician might then say, "What you just did — that's how you say the [t] sound."

[p] and [b]

The following techniques facilitate production of [p]. To facilitate [b], follow the same steps, but also instruct the client to turn on the voice box.

PHONETIC PLACEMENT

Method:

1. Ask the client to blow out a long breath.
2. Next, instruct the client to use his or her lips to break up the breath into shorter and shorter bursts. If additional assistance is needed, manually close the client's mouth. [p] results as the client quickly opens and closes his or her lips while continuing to emit a long breath.

SHAPING

[p] from [b] (***Final Consonant Devoicing)

First Method: Instruct the client to turn off his or her "voice box," which for some clients is sufficient instruction to result in [p]. Another possible instruction is to tell the client that, "We don't want the voice — we just want the air."

Second Method: Demonstrate the contrast between [b] and [p]. Alternatively, if the client is able to make a voicing contrast between other consonants (such as between [t] and [d]), draw attention to those contrasts. For some clients this is sufficient to result in [p].

[p] from [p̬]

Method: Use a mirror to demonstrate the difference between [p] and [p̬]. In more severe cases, press up the client's lower lip using a finger or a tongue depressor until the lower lip is in contact with upper lip, which results in [p]. (*Note:* To facilitate [b], develop from [b̬]).

[p] from [ɸ]

Method: Use a mirror to demonstrate the difference between [p] and [ɸ]. In more severe cases, press the client's lips together with your fingers, which results in [p]. (*Note:* To facilitate [b], develop from [β]).

[m]

[m] is facilitated similarly to [p] and [b], except for the addition of nasality.

PHONETIC PLACEMENT

Nasality

First Method:

1. The clinician and client practice taking turns breathing out with their mouths closed, using a piece of paper or a mirror placed under their noses to draw attention to airflow.

2. Next, contrast nasal and oral airflow by placing a piece of paper or a mirror in front of the client's mouth while the client produces an oral consonant such as [b] or [d].

3. Ask the client to attempt [b] with his or her lips closed, but with the voice box vibrating and air coming out the nose. This often results in [m].

Second Method:

1 The clinician and client begin by taking a deep breath, holding it, and letting the air out through the nose. This results in a voiceless [m].

2. Next, have the client practice saying [ɑ].

3. The clinician and client alternate taking a deep breath while holding their noses and then letting air out through the nose while saying "ah" with the mouth closed, which results in [m].

SHAPING

[m] from [b]

Method: Instruct the client to produce [b] followed by a schwa with his or her mouth closed and with air coming out the nose. If needed, a mirror or piece of paper placed under the nostrils may be used to increase the client's awareness of air flowing from the nose. This often results in correct production of [m].

[w]

PHONETIC PLACEMENT

Method:

1. Ask the client to round his or her lips and to place them close together. If the lips are too close or too far apart, move them in to the correct position with a finger or a tongue depressor.

2. Next, instruct the client to raise (or hump up) the very back of his or her tongue toward the roof of the mouth. If needed, push the tongue back with a tongue depressor.

3. Instruct the client to breathe out with his or her voice box on, which often results in [wu].

SHAPING

[w] from [u]

Method:

1. Ask the client to say [u].

2. Next, while the client says [u], ask him or her to almost close the lips, resulting in [w]. (If needed, the client's lips can be moved manually to the appropriate position.)

[w] from [b]

First Method:

Instruct the client to open his or her lips and pucker them slightly while saying [bu], resulting in [wu].

Second Method:

1. Instruct the client to say [u] + [ɑ] several times as rapidly as possible, resulting in [uwɑ].

2. After [uwɑ] is established, instruct the client to "make the [u] silent," which results in [wɑ].

[f] and [v]

The following techniques facilitate [f]. To facilitate [v], follow the same steps, but also instruct the client to turn on the voice box.

PHONETIC PLACEMENT

Method: Instruct the client to touch his or her lower lip with the bottom of the upper front teeth and then to blow, which often results in [f]. In more severe cases, move the client's lip to the correct position using a finger or a tongue depressor. Alternately, instruct the client to "bite" the lower lip with the upper teeth and then to blow.

SHAPING

[f] from [v] (***Final Consonant Devoicing)

Method: Instruct the client to say [v] and then turn off the voice box. This often is sufficient to result in [f]. (*Note:* To facilitate [v], shape from [f] and instruct the client to turn on the voice box.)

[f] from [p] (***Stopping)

Method:

1. Say [f] and [p] to demonstrate the difference between bilabial and labio-dental places of production.

2. Instruct the client to say [p] and then instruct him or her to retract the lower lip until the upper teeth are in contact with the lower lip.

3. Instruct the client to separate his or her teeth and lips slightly, resulting in [f]. (*Note:* To facilitate [v], develop from [b].)

[f] from [a]

Method:

1. Instruct the client to say [a].

2. Place the client's lower lip under the edge of his or her upper front teeth.

3. Next, instruct the client to blow air out between his or her lips and teeth so that friction is audible. (In more severe cases, move the client's lips to the correct position and instruct the client to blow out.)

4. Instruct the client to turn off the voice box, resulting in [f]. (*Note:* To facilitate [v], do not instruct the client to turn off the voice, since [a] and [v] are both voiced sounds.)

[θ] and [ð]

The following techniques facilitate [θ]. To facilitate [ð], follow the same steps but also instruct the client to turn on the voice box.

PHONETIC PLACEMENT

First Method:

1. Demonstrate placing the tongue between the upper and lower front teeth.

2. Place a feather or small piece of paper in front of the client's mouth, and instruct the client to blow through the teeth to make the object move, resulting in [θ].

Second Method:

1. Place a tongue depressor in front of the client's mouth, instructing the client to touch the depressor with his or her tongue tip.

2. When the client's tongue is out, gently push up the client's lower jaw so that his or her teeth and tongue come into contact.

3. Instruct the client to blow over the tongue. If the client is only able to produce an interdental [t], gently insert a Q-tip between the client's tongue tip and upper teeth to create a sufficiently broad opening to allow continuous airflow. This often results in [θ].

SHAPING

[θ] from [ð] (***Final Consonant Devoicing)

Method: Instruct the client to say [ð] and then ask him or her to turn off the voice box, resulting in [θ]. (*Note:* To facilitate [ð], instruct the client to turn on the voice while saying [θ].)

[θ] from [f]

Method:

1. Demonstrate the difference between the place of production for [f] and the place of production for [θ].

2. Next, instruct the client to say [f] while moving his or her tongue to lie between the upper and lower front teeth, resulting in [θ]. (*Note:* To facilitate [ð], develop from [v].)

[θ] from [s]

Method:

1. Demonstrate the difference between the place of production for [s] and the place of production for [θ].

2. Next, instruct the client to say [s] while moving his or her tongue to lie between the upper and lower front teeth, resulting in [θ]. (*Note:* To facilitate [ð], develop from [z].)

[t] and [d]

The following techniques facilitate [t]. To facilitate [d], follow the same steps but also instruct the client to turn on the voice box.

PHONETIC PLACEMENT

First Method:

1. Use a mirror as a visual aid to instruct the client to press his or her tongue tip against the bump behind the front teeth.

2. Instruct the client to lower the tongue quickly. If needed, a piece of paper or the client's hand placed in front of the mouth may help direct the client to the plosive release of the sound, which often results in a sound that approximates [t].

Second Method:

1. The clinician demonstrates by placing a tongue depressor under his or her tongue and then under the client's tongue. The tongue depressor serves as a shelf for the tongue, which is then raised to be even with the bottom of the upper teeth.

2. Next, raise the client's tongue on the shelf and ask the client to touch "the bump" rapidly with his or her tongue tip. If needed, a piece of paper or the client's hand placed in front of the mouth may help direct the client to the plosive release of the sound. This often results in a sound approximating [t]. (*Note:* To facilitate [d], instruct the client to turn on the voice.)

SHAPING

[t] from [d] (***Final Consonant Devoicing)

Method: Instruct the client to say [d] and then turn off the voice box. For some clients, this is sufficient instruction to result in [t]. (*Note:* To facilitate [d], instruct the client to turn on the voice while saying [t].)

[t] from [p]

Method:

1. Instruct the client to say [p] + schwa.

2. Ask the client to place his or her tongue tip between the lips and to say [p] + schwa again.

3. Next, ask the client to make "a sound almost like [p]" by making contact between his or her tongue tip and upper lip.

4. Instruct the client to make contact between the tongue tip and "the bump," resulting in [t]. (*Note:* To facilitate [d], develop from [b].)

[n]

[n] is facilitated similarly to [t] and [d], except for the addition of nasality.

PHONETIC PLACEMENT

Method:

1. The clinician and client take turns breathing out with their mouths closed and with the tongue in position for [d].

2. Next, place a piece of paper or a mirror under the client's nose to draw attention to air coming out the nose, then contrast this to placing a piece of paper or a mirror in front of the mouth when producing an oral consonant such as [b] or [d].

3. Ask the client to attempt [d] with his or her lips closed but with the voice box vibrating and air coming out the nose. This often results in [n].

SHAPING

[n] from [d]

Method: Instruct the client to take a deep breath, hold it with the tongue in position for [d], close the mouth, and then let the air out through his or her nose, resulting in [n].

[s] and [z]

The following techniques facilitate [s]. To facilitate [z], follow the same steps but also instruct the client to turn on the voice box.

---

[s] Up or [s] Down?

Some people produce [s] and [z] with the tongue tip up behind the upper front teeth, others say them with the tongue tip down behind the lower front teeth. Neither one is the "right way." Follow the client's lead in deciding which way to teach [s] and [z]. If the client appears to find it easier to say [s] and [z] with the tongue tip up, teach the sounds that way; if the client appears to find it easier to say [s] and [z] with the tongue tip down, teach the sounds that way.

PHONETIC PLACEMENT

First Method (tongue tip up or down):

1. Place a tongue depressor just behind the client's upper or lower front teeth and ask the client to use his or her tongue tip to hold it there.
2. Next, ask the client to keep his or her tongue still while the clinician carefully removes the tongue depressor.
3. Ask the client to breathe out, resulting in [s].

Second Method (tongue tip up or down):

1. Instruct the client to place the tip of his or her tongue behind either the upper or lower front teeth and then ask the client to pull the tongue away a little bit.
2. Close the client's teeth so the teeth are barely touching.
3. Place a finger in front of the center of the client's mouth, saying "Blow air slowly over your tongue toward my finger." The sound produced by the client when he or she blows out approximates [s].

Third Method (tongue tip up):

1. Make a shelf by placing a tongue depressor against the lower edges of the client's upper teeth.

2. Next, ask the client to place his or her tongue on the shelf. If needed, place a tongue depressor under the client's tongue tip to bring the "elevator up" so that the tongue depressor touches the lower front teeth.

3. Ask the client to breathe out through his or her mouth. The resulting sound approximates [s].

Fourth Method (tongue tip up):

1. Instruct the client to raise his or her tongue so that the sides are firmly in contact with the inner surface of the upper back teeth. An alternate method is to instruct the client to stick out his or her tongue slightly, lower the upper teeth to come into contact with the sides of the tongue, and then pull the tongue inside his or her mouth.

2. Ask the client to groove the tongue slightly along the midline. If needed, ask the client to protrude the tongue and place a clean object such as a drinking straw along the midline of the tongue. Then ask the client to raise the sides of the tongue slightly around the straw.

3. Carefully withdraw the straw.

4. Ask the client to place the tip of his or her tongue about a quarter of an inch behind the upper teeth and then ask the client to bring the teeth together.

5. Instruct the client to blow air along the groove of the tongue toward the lower teeth. If the client has difficulty directing the air along the tongue groove, insert a drinking straw into the client's mouth and instruct the client to blow through the straw, which often results in [s].

Fifth Method (tongue tip down):

1. Instruct the client to brush his or her lower gums with the tongue while attempting to say [s].

2. Ask the client to stop moving his or her tongue and to bring the upper and lower teeth close together, but not touching.

3. Instruct the client to breathe out through the mouth, resulting in [s].

SHAPING (tongue tip up or down)

[s] from [z] (***Final Consonant Devoicing)

Method: Instruct the client to say [z] and then to turn off the voice box. For some clients, this is sufficient instruction to result in [s]. (*Note:* To facilitate [z], instruct the client to turn on the voice while saying [s].)

[s] from [θ] (***Lisping)

Method:

1. Instruct the client to protrude his or her tongue between the teeth and to say [θ].

2. As client says [θ], instruct him or her to bring the tongue back into the mouth and behind the upper or lower front teeth, depending on which variety of [s] is being facilitated. An alternate method is to ask the client to scrape his or her tongue tip back along the back of the front teeth. (If needed, the tip of the client's tongue can be pushed inward with a tongue depressor.)

3. Next, ask the client to either raise or lower the tongue tip slightly, depending on which type of [s] is being taught.

4. Ask the client to blow air through the mouth, which typically results in [s]. (*Note:* To facilitate [z], develop from [ð].)

[s] from [ɬ] (***Lateralization)

First Method:

1. Demonstrate air flowing through a straw protruding from the side of the mouth when a lateral [s] is made and air flowing through a straw placed in the front of the mouth when a correct [s] is made.

2. Encourage the client to close his or her teeth and to direct the airflow through a straw placed in front of the mouth. This typically results in [s]. (*Note:* To facilitate [z], develop from lateral [z]).

Second Method:

1. Instruct the client to produce a lateral [s] [ɬ].

2. Draw imaginary circles with a Q-tip where the groove should occur in the center of the tongue to indicate to the client where the air should flow during [s].

3. Next, draw a small circle on a piece of paper and hold it in front of the client's mouth at the point where air should be emitted if the air flows over the top of the tongue.

4. Instruct the client to direct the air through the circle while saying [s]. An alternate method is to instruct the client to use his or her fingers instead of paper. If the client's fingers are used, the sensation of air is felt more keenly if the client's fingers are wet. (*Note:* To facilitate [z], develop from lateral [z].)

[s] from [t] (***Stopping)

First Method:

1. Instruct the client to say [t] in "tea" with strong aspiration. If said quickly and forcefully, [tsi] should result. As an alternative to this procedure, ask the client to say [tsi] instead of "tea."

2. Instruct the client to say [tsi] without the vowel, resulting in [ts].

3. Ask the client to prolong the [s] portion of [ts], resulting in tsss.

4. Ask the client to make [t] silent, resulting in [s].

Second Method:

1. Ask the client to open his or her mouth and to put the tongue in position for [t].

2. Instruct the client to drop his or her tongue slightly and to send the air over the tongue. Place the client's finger in front of the mouth to feel the emission of air. The resulting sound is [s].

[s] from [ʃ]

Method:

1. Instruct the client to say [ʃ].

2. Ask the client to retract his or her lips into a smile. Often, this results in the tongue moving forward slightly into the position for [s]. If needed, however, instruct the client to move the tongue slightly forward. The resulting sound is [s]. (*Note:* To facilitate [z], develop from [ʒ], or instruct the client to turn on his or her voice box.)

[s] from [d] (***Stopping and ***Prevocalic Voicing)

Method:

1. Ask the client to place his or her tongue in position for [d].

2. Instruct the client to release the tongue a little bit and to force the air over the tongue.

3. Ask the client to turn off the voice. The sound that results when the client turns off the voice is [s]. (*Note:* To facilitate [z], develop from [d] or use [s] and instruct the client to turn on his or her voice box.)

[s] from [i]

Method:

1. Instruct the client to say [i].

2. Ask the client to turn off his or her voice and gradually close the teeth until [s] results (*Note:* To facilitate [z], instruct the client to keep the voice box on.)

[s] from [h]

Method:

1. Instruct the client to gradually close the teeth while saying [h].

2. Ask the client to raise his or her tongue tip gradually while producing a prolonged [h] until the resulting sound is [s]. (*Note:* To facilitate [z], instruct the client to turn on the voice.)

[s] from [f]

Method:

1. Instruct the client to lift his or her tongue tip slowly while making a prolonged [f].

2. Ask the client to bring the front teeth close together but not quite touching. If needed, gently pull out the client's lower lip slightly.

3. Ask the client to smile while making the sound, resulting in [s]. (*Note:* To facilitate [z], develop from [v] or use [s] and instruct the client to turn on his or her voice box.)

[l]

PHONETIC PLACEMENT

First Method:

1. Touch the client's alveolar ridge with a tongue depressor, peanut butter, or lollipop to indicate the place of production for [l].

2. Ask the client to place his or her tongue tip in the place indicated, to relax, and to let air flow out from the sides of the tongue. The resulting sound is voiceless [l].

3. Instruct the client to turn on the voice box, resulting in [l].

Second Method:

1. Place a straw midline on the client's tongue groove to demonstrate central air emission. Ask the client to blow out onto an open hand or a piece of paper. An alternative (or additional) demonstration of central air emission is to ask the client to prepare his or her mouth to say [s] but to breathe in. Cool air is felt midline on the upper tongue surface.

2. Next, place a straw in each corner of the client's mouth. Ask the client to breathe out into his or her open hand or on a piece of paper. If an additional demonstration is needed, remove the straws and ask the client to breathe in and to feel the cool air on the sides of the tongue over which the air is emitted. To demonstrate the feel of the air more vividly, ask the client to suck on a piece of peppermint candy for a few minutes before performing the demonstration.

3. After lateral emission of air is obtained, ask the client to place his or her tongue tip in contact with the roof of the mouth behind the upper front teeth and to blow out over the sides of the tongue. If needed, place straws in the side of the client's mouth while the tongue tip is held in contact with the roof of the mouth.

4. Then instruct the client to blow air out the side straws, which results in voiceless [l].

5. Voicing is obtained by asking the client to turn on the voice box. The resulting sound is [l].

Third Method:

1. Place a tongue depressor under the client's tongue tip and raise the tongue tip behind the upper front teeth.

2. Ask the client to say [l] while maintaining contact between the tongue tip and the roof of the mouth. The resulting sound is [l].

Fourth Method ([l] in consonant clusters):

Instruct the client to place the tongue in the position for [l] before initiating the cluster, resulting in a consonant cluster containing [l].

SHAPING

[l] from [θ] or [ð]

Method:

1. Instruct the client to place the tongue tip between the teeth as for [θ].

2. Lower the client's jaw.

3. Instruct the client to slowly draw the tongue tip backward but to keep the tongue tip in contact with the back of the teeth and the ridge behind the two front teeth.

4. Next, instruct the client to say [l], being sure that contact between the tongue and the roof of the mouth is maintained.

[l] from [i] or [u]

Method:

1. Instruct the client to open his or her mouth wide as for [ɑ] but to raise the tongue as for [i].

2. Ask the client to keep the tongue up as for [i] but to say [ɑ], resulting in a light (alveolar) [l]. (*Note:* For a dark [velar] [l], follow the same steps but ask the client to say [u] instead of [i].)

[ɚ]

PHONETIC PLACEMENT

First Method (retroflex or humped):

Instruct the client to growl like a tiger ([gɚ]). Alternately, ask the client to make the "arm wrestling sound" ([ɚ]) while arm wrestling with the clinician.

Second Method (retroflex or humped):

Instruct the client to lie on his or her back, relax the mouth, and say [ɚ].

Third Method (humped):

1. Instruct the client to lower his or her tongue tip.

2. Ask the client to hump up the back of the tongue as for "a silent [k]."

3. Ask the client to make the sides of the back of the tongue touch the insides of the back teeth.

4. Ask the client to turn on the voice box, resulting in [ɚ].

SHAPING

[ɚ] (humped) From [w] (***Gliding)

Method:

1. Lower the client's jaw slightly.

2. Ask the client to say [w] but to "let the lips go to sleep." An alternate method is to tell the client, "No kissing frogs" to prompt an unround lip position. If needed, push the client's lips back with a tongue depressor to an unrounded position.

3. While reminding the client to keep the lips asleep, instruct him or her to make the tongue position for [d].

4. Ask the client to retract the tongue slightly while lowering the tongue tip and to say [ɚ].

[ɚ] (retroflex) from [ð]

Method:

1. Instruct the client to place his or her tongue as for [ð].

2. Ask the client to quickly draw the tongue tip back and slightly up, which typically results in [ɚ].

[ɚ] (humped) from [d]

Method: Lower the client's jaw slightly as for [d]. While the client's jaw is lowered, ask him or her to pull back the tongue slightly, to lower the tongue tip, and to say [ɚ].

[ɚ] (retroflex) from [ʃ]

Method:

1. Instruct the client to say [ʃ], but to curl the tongue tip back while keeping contact with the tongue on the insides of the back teeth.

2. Ask the client to turn on the voice box, resulting in [ɚ].

[ɚ] (retroflex) from [l]

Method:

1. Lower the client's jaw slightly and instruct the client to say [l] + [ə].

2. While the client says [l] + [ə], instruct him or her to curl back the tongue tip back until [ɚ] results. (If needed, a tongue depressor can be used to push the tongue back.)

[ɚ] from [ɑ]

Method:

1. Instruct the client to say "ah."

2. Next, ask the client to raise his or her tongue slightly toward the roof of the mouth and say [ɑr]. (If needed, instruct the client to raise the tongue tip or to raise his or her tongue slightly and to say [ɑ] forcibly.) The resulting sound is [ɑr].

[ɚ] (retroflex) from [i]

Method:

1. Instruct the client to say [i].

2. While the client is saying [i], ask him or her to lift the tongue and curl back the tongue tip to say [ɚ].

[r]

PHONETIC PLACEMENT

First Method:

Instruct the client to make a sound like a motor starting up ([rɚ]).

Second Method:

1. Ask the client to place his or her tongue tip behind the upper front teeth. (If needed, place the client's tongue tip on a shelf made with a tongue depressor.)

2. Next, ask the client to curl the tongue backward without touching the roof of the mouth until it cannot go back farther.

3. Lower the client's jaw slightly and instruct the client to say [ru].

Facilitation of [r]

With some clients, correct production of [ɚ] generalizes to [r] without the need for treatment.

SHAPING

[r] from [ɚ]

Method:

1. Ask the client to say [ɚ].

2. Next, ask the client to say [ɚ] followed by [i] or some other vowel.

3. Instruct the client to say [ɚi] several times as quickly as possible, resulting in [ɚri]. After [ri] is established, instruct the client to say [ɚ] silently, resulting in [ri].

[tʃ] and [dʒ]

The following techniques facilitate [tʃ]. To facilitate [dʒ], follow the same steps, but also instruct the client to turn on the voice box.

PHONETIC PLACEMENT

Method:

1. Ask the client to pucker the lips slightly.

2. Ask the client to make the tongue tip touch "the bump" behind the two upper front teeth.

3. Next, instruct the client to make the sneezing sound (choo!) while keeping the lips slightly puckered and the tongue tip on the alveolar ridge. If [ts] results, instruct the client to move the tongue tip back slightly while maintaining contact with the roof of the mouth, resulting in [tʃ].

SHAPING

[tʃ] from [ʃ]

Method: Instruct the client to say a quick [ʃ] with the tongue tip touching "the bump," resulting in [tʃ]. (*Note:* To facilitate [dʒ], develop from [ʒ].)

[tʃ] from [t] or [ʃ]

Method:

1. Explain that [tʃ] is [t] and [ʃ] said together very quickly.

2. Next, ask the client to say [ʃ].

3. Instruct the client to say [t] and then to draw the tongue tip back a little and say [t] again.

4. With the client's tongue tip in the position for the "back" [t], instruct the client to quickly say [t] followed by [ʃ], resulting in [tʃ]. (*Note:* To facilitate [dʒ], develop from [d] and [ʒ].)

[ʃ] and [ʒ]

The following techniques facilitate [ʃ]. To facilitate [ʒ], follow the same steps but also instruct the client to turn on the voice box.

PHONETIC PLACEMENT

Method:

1. Ask the client to part his or her teeth and lips.

2. Touch the client's tongue just behind the tip with a tongue depressor. Instruct the client to move the place just touched to the roof of the mouth behind the "bumpy part." (If needed, a tongue depressor may be used to push the tongue back from the upper front teeth.)

3. Next, instruct the client to lower the tongue slightly. (If needed, direct the tongue down slightly with a tongue depressor.)

4. Ask the client to hold this position, pucker his or her lips slightly, and breathe out through the mouth, which results in [ʃ].

SHAPING

[ʃ] from [ʒ] (***Final Consonant Devoicing)

Method: Instruct the client to say [ʒ] and then turn off the voice, resulting in [ʃ]. (*Note:* To facilitate [ʒ], instruct the client to turn on the voice while saying [ʃ].

[ʃ] from [s] (***Fronting)

Method: Ask the client to say [s]. While the client is saying [s], instruct him or her to pucker the lips slightly and to draw the tongue back a little until [ʃ] results.

[ʃ] from [i] or [ɑ]

Method:

1. Instruct the client to say [i] or [ɑ], first with the voice on and then with the voice off.

2. Next, ask the client to pucker the lips slightly.

3. Raise the client's lower jaw slightly.

4. Ask the client to breathe out silently while raising the tongue, resulting in [ʃ].

[j]

PHONETIC PLACEMENT

Method:

1. Instruct the client to place the tongue flat in the mouth. (If needed, gently press down the tongue with a tongue depressor.)

2. Open the client's mouth and gently tap the middle portion of the tongue, asking the client to slightly raise the place you touched.

3. Ask the client to breathe out with the voice on, resulting in [j].

SHAPING

[j] from [ʒ]

Method: Instruct the client to say [ʒ] several times quickly. Often, this results in [j]. An additional cue is to ask the client to lower the tongue slightly.

[k] and [g]

The following techniques facilitate [k]. To facilitate [g], follow the same steps but also instruct the client to turn on the voice box.

PHONETIC PLACEMENT

First Method:

1. Instruct the client to place a hand in contact with the underside of your mouth.

2. While holding the client's chin stationary, direct the client's attention to the muscle movements that occur as you repeat [k] several times.

3. Ask the client to imitate you, resulting in [k].

Second Method:

Ask the client to drop his or her head back and say [ku], which sometimes is sufficient to result in [k].

Third Method:

Ask the client to pretend to cough up a fish bone from the throat. Alternately, ask the client to imitate you while you pretend to shoot a gun, resulting in [ku ku ku].

Fourth Method:

1. Press your hand underneath the client's chin near the juncture of the jaw and neck where [k] is produced.

2. Instruct the client to whisper [ku] as you release the pressure, resulting in a soft [k].

Fifth Method:

1. Ask the client to place the tongue tip behind the lower front teeth. (If needed, a tongue depressor may be used to keep the tongue in place.)

2. Ask the client to hump the back of the tongue and say [ku].

SHAPING

[k] from [t] (***Fronting)

Method:

1. Ask the client to place the tongue tip behind the two lower front teeth while making [t]. (If needed, the tongue tip may be held down with a tongue depressor.)

2. Next, ask the client to hump up the back of the tongue and say [k]. (*Note:* For [g], shape from [d].)

[k] from [g] (***Final Consonant Devoicing)

Method: Instruct the client to say [g] and then to turn off the voice box. For some clients, this is sufficient instruction to result in [k]. (*Note:* To facilitate [g], instruct the client to turn on the voice while saying [k].)

[k] from [i]

Method:

1. Instruct the client to say [i].

2. Next, ask the client to say a long [i] but to raise up the back of the tongue as the vowel ends, resulting in [k]. If needed, instruct the client to turn off the voice. (*Note:* To facilitate [g], do not ask the client to turn off the voice.)

[ŋ]

[ŋ] is facilitated similarly to [k] and [g] except for the addition of nasality.

PHONETIC PLACEMENT

Method:

1. Ask the client to breathe out with his or her mouth closed.

2. Next, place a piece of paper or a mirror under the client's nose, drawing attention to air coming out the nose. Contrast this with placing a piece of paper or a mirror in front of the client's mouth while producing an oral consonant such as [b] or [d].

3. Ask the client to attempt [g] with the lips closed, voice box vibrating, and air coming out the nose, resulting in [ŋ].

SHAPING

None recommended.

[h]

PHONETIC PLACEMENT

First Method: Instruct the client to practice blowing out a candle, resulting in [h].

Second Method: To produce [h] in conjunction with a vowel, ask the client to say a vowel and then to blow out the vowel that follows [h], resulting in [h] + vowel.

SHAPING

None typically is required.

CHAPTER

6

Options in Assessment and Treatment

The following topics are discussed in this chapter:

I. OVERVIEW

This chapter summarizes many of the major care options presented in previous chapters. Case studies of clients are presented to illustrate similarities and differences in providing care at four stages in articulation and phonological development. Each client is a composite of several real clients seen either by the author or his colleagues. Finally, the "boxes" in this chapter offer questions and describe promising avenues for future directions in treatment.

II. MAJOR CARE OPTIONS FOR CLIENTS IN STAGE 1

A. The Client: Bill

Bill was born with Down syndrome, a genetic disorder occurring in approximately 1 in 700 births. Children with Down syndrome typically are moderately retarded and suffer from heart conditions, weak muscle tone, and respiratory problems. The first months at home Bill developed slowly but steadily, although he was a difficult child to feed. Bill underwent heart surgery at 6 months of age to correct a faulty heart valve, and during that time in the hospital, he appeared to regress in some of his earlier developmental gains. Bill was referred to a speech-language clinician when he was 10 months of age.

B. Legal Basis of Care (Chapter 1)

Bill was eligible to be considered for articulation and phonological care under provisions of PL 99–457, which provides legal protection to children with diagnosed developmental delays and children at high risk for future developmental delays. PL 99–457 also gives discretion to the individual states to decide whether to develop laws to protect children with conditions that place them at-risk for future developmental difficulties. Importantly, even if Bill was not delayed in development, he is eligible to receive developmental services, because the law recognizes that Down syndrome is a genetic disorder which places Bill at high risk for future developmental delays.

Syllables and Words

Nearly all speech-language clinicians know that sounds can be decomposed into bundles of distinctive features. Much less is known about the structure of syllables and words,

---

largely because generative phonology (the linguistic theory which historically has had the greatest influence on speech-language pathology) never concerned itself with them. Generative phonology is gone now, largely replaced by two new theories — autosegmental phonology and metrical phonology, both of which give central roles to the structures of syllables and words. Several investigators are exploring the possible clinical benefits of autosegmental and metrical phonology for treating articulation and phonological disorders (Bernhardt, in press; Bernhardt & Gilbert, 1992; Bernhardt & Stoel-Gammon, in press; Schwartz, 1992). If the results of these studies meet their early promise, in the future clinicians may be as familiar with such syllable- and word-level concepts as onsets, rimes, moras, and tiers as we are today with sound and sound class concepts such as manner of production, place of production, and distinctive features.

C. Screening and Assessment (Chapter 2)

The assessment consisted of three steps: an initial observation, collection of a sample of vocalizations, and hypothesis testing. The assessment began by talking with Bill's caregivers and observing Bill at rest in his mother's arms. To obtain a sample of vocalizations, the clinician's options were either to elicit vocalizations or to ask one of Bill's caregivers to perform this function. In almost all cases, a caregiver elicits vocalizations more easily from an infant than someone less familiar with the client's habits and likes, so the clinician chose to have Bill's parents act as the elicitors. Hypotheses raised during the initial evaluation session were addressed during subsequent treatment sessions.

1. **Sample Size.** The clinician obtained 10 vocalizations during the initial assessment and 14 more during the elicitation portion of subsequent treatment sessions. Although not a large sample, it was deemed sufficient to begin treatment.

2. **Transcription System.** The clinician's options were to transcribe and record Bill's vocalizations or to utilize a check mark system such as that presented in Appendix 3J. The clinician elected to use the check mark system.

3. **Types of Speech Samples.** The clinician's options were spontaneous speech, elicited speech, or a combination of both. Bill's level of development precluded all but spontaneous speech.

4. **Elicitation Activities.** The following objects were available to elicit vocalizations: a mirror, bubbles, pop-up toys, manipulable toys, a toy drum, and several toy cars.

5. **Options for Published Assessment Instruments.** None.

6. **Related Assessments.** In addition to the articulation and phonological assessment, the clinician performed a parent interview, a hearing screening, a complete language evaluation, and an oral-mechanism evaluation.

D. Analysis (Chapter 3)

The following options were considered (the order of assessments reflects their presentation in Chapter 3 and does not reflect the order in which they were performed):

Severity

Age norms

Better abilities

Related analyses

1. **Severity.** The principle clinical options were calculation of percentage of development and severity rating scales such as those presented in Chapter 3. The clinician selected a severity rating scale. The results indicated that Bill was severely delayed in vocal development compared to both his language reception abilities and chronological age.

2. **Age Norms.** The clinical option was analysis of prespeech vocalizations. Results of the assessment indicated that Bill's vocalizations approximated those of an infant near 1 to 2 months of age. The clinician also noted that one instance of cooing (a back vowel) was observed.

3. **Better Abilities.** The clinical option was stimulability. Results of this analysis indicated that Bill was unstimulable for any type of vocalization.

4. **Related Analyses.** The clinical options were adjusted age and developmental age. Because Bill was not born prematurely, adjusted age was not calculated. Results of the language evaluation indicated that Bill's language reception and play abilities approximated those of an infant near 6 months of age.

E. Treatment (Chapter 4)

Bill was accepted into treatment as an outpatient in a hospital-based early intervention program.

1. **Purpose.** Articulation and phonological care focused on facilitating the acquisition of vocal skills that underlie later speech development.

2. **Long-term Goals.** The long-term treatment goal for Bill was for his articulation and phonological development to be commensurate to his developmental age. A second long-term treatment goal was to facilitate parent education and training.

3. **Short-term Goals.** The options for short-term goals were to increase Bill's opportunities to vocalize and to facilitate the acquisition of developmentally advanced vocalizations. The first goal might have been selected if Bill was hospitalized or suffering from neglect, because in those situations providing regular opportunities to play and vocalize sometimes is sufficient to result in impressive developmental changes. However, because Bill was delayed in vocal development despite many opportunities to vocalize, the clinician chose the second option.

4. **Selecting Treatment Targets.** The clinician considered behaviors in advance of Bill's present level of vocal development. Syllables containing back consonants and vowels were given the highest consideration, because during the evaluation, Bill produced one instance of cooing, showing that the behavior — although infrequent — was within Bill's vocal capacities.

5. **Most and Least Knowledge Methods.** The options were to select treatment targets slightly or substantially in advance of Bill's present vocal abilities. In the vast majority of cases, infants progress by small steps in vocal development, and so, perforce, the most knowledge method was selected.

6. **Number of Treatment Targets.** The treatment options were to train wide or deep. Training wide was selected because this choice seemed better suited to Bill's cognitive and developmental abilities.

7. **Changing Treatment Targets.** The clinician's options were flexibility, time, and percentage. A flexible approach was selected because it seemed better suited to Bill's level of cognitive development. The clinician, for example, arrived at each treatment session prepared to facilitate a variety of back consonants and back vowels; the exact choice of the session's treatment target was based on the sounds that Bill was willing to attempt.

8. **Linguistic Level to Introduce Treatment Targets.** This option was not pertinent to Bill's care.

F. Administrative Decisions (Chapter 4)

The administrative options involved session length, group or individual care, length of individual treatment activities, and types of activities. The clinician elected to facilitate vocal development in a group that met four times a week for 30 minutes a session Ten minutes was devoted primarily to stimulating vocal and language development. All of the activities involved play, and individual vocal stimulation activities lasted from a few seconds to a few minutes. Bill's parents were encouraged to participate in group activities. Additional counseling of parents regarding vocal development was provided in individual weekly meetings.

G. Facilitative Techniques (Chapter 5)

The clinician's primary options for facilitative techniques were motherese and, occasionally, imitation. Language was stimulated simultaneously with vocal development.

Throughout the session, the clinician and Bill engaged in routines that had been found to encourage Bill to vocalize. While playing, the clinician occasionally produced vocalizations for Bill to imitate. If Bill imitated the vocalization, that utterance became the treatment target for the next few minutes as the clinician and Bill engaged in reciprocal vocalizations. If, however, Bill produced a different vocalization, that became the treatment target for the next few minutes. The clinician praised and looked excited when Bill produced any type of vocalization; when Bill cooed, the clinician praised him even more.

H. Assessing Clinical Progress (Chapter 4)

The clinician's primary options were pre- and post-tests, ongoing information gathering, and parent questionnaires. The clinician assessed treatment progress using the vocal development checklist (Appendix 3J) and a severity scale as pre- and post-tests. A parent interview designed to ascertain both the family's knowledge of vocal development and their degree of satisfaction with Bill's therapeutic progress was also undertaken. Results of the post-tests indicated good clinical progress; Bill's family demonstrated increased knowledge of vocal development in response to questions asked by the clinician and they expressed satisfaction with their son's clinical progress.

Literacy

Webster and Plante (1992) and Hodson (1994) have observed that at least some children with articulation and phonological disorders also demonstrate limited skills in phonological awareness (awareness of segments within words). This is an intriguing observation because phonological awareness is thought to be a good predictor of later success in reading and spelling. Persons showing less developed phonological awareness skills also demonstrate less ability in literacy skilly (Goswami & Bryant, 1990; Maclean, Bryant, & Bradley, 1987). This raises two intriguing questions: Should children with articulation and phonological disorders be considered at risk for future problems in reading and spelling? Should appropriate clients receive treatment to facilitate phonological awareness?

III. MAJOR CARE OPTIONS FOR CLIENTS IN STAGE 2

A. The Client: Mary

Mary was born 2 months prematurely, but she did not experience overt medical complications resulting from her prematurity and was discharged from the hospital shortly after her original due date, small but healthy. It was explained to Mary's family, however, that she was at risk for future developmental problems due to possible damage to her immature neurological system. Mary was referred to a speech-language clinician at 23 months of age.

B. Legal Basis of Care (Chapter 1)

Like Bill, Mary was eligible to receive articulation and phonological care under provisions of PL 99–457 (Part H), which provides legal protection to children with developmental delays in (1) cognition, physical skills, communication, or psychosocial development and (2) children with physical or mental conditions that place them at high probability for future developmental delays, including fetal alcohol syndrome, seizure disorders, and chromosomal abnormalities such as Down syndrome. The law gives discretion to the individual states to decide whether to develop laws to protect children with conditions that place them at risk for future developmental difficulties, including very low birthweight resulting from prematurity, respiratory distress, and asphyxia. It should be noted that, even if Mary was not delayed in development, she would have been eligible to receive developmental services in many states, because the law recognizes that prematurity places children at risk for future developmental delays.

Group Therapy and Parent Involvement

Phonogroup: A Practical Guide to Enhancing Phonological Remediation (Kelman & Edwards, 1994) is an extremely practical and well-written guide to providing group therapy and promoting parent involvement. The intended populations for intervention are preschoolers and younger school-aged children. I mention *Phonogroup* here because, although group therapy and parent involvement are not new ideas, the book addresses an important topic that is likely to continue to grow more important as the increasing number of clients needing help forces clinicians to be ever more effective and efficient.

C. Assessment (Chapter 2)

The assessment consisted of three steps: initial observation, collection of the speech sample, and hypothesis testing. The assessment began by observing Mary while she and her mother played. The clinical options for collecting the speech sample were for the clinician or Mary's mother to act as the elicitor. The clinician chose the latter option, because in almost all cases, a caregiver elicits speech from a toddler more easily than someone unfamiliar with the child's likes and dislikes. Hypotheses raised about Mary's speech during the initial evaluation were pursued during subsequent treatment sessions. Gradually, the clinician became the elicitor as the clinician and Mary grew more comfortable with each other.

1. **Sample Size.** A speech sample of 50 to 100 utterances, which is often obtained with older children, is seldom feasible with most toddlers, especially those under 18 months of age. The clinician obtained a total of 13 different renditions of 10 different words on the first day of evaluation, and an additional 9 different renditions of 4 additional words were obtained over subsequent evaluations undertaken concurrent with the onset of treatment.

2. **Transcription System.** The clinician transcribed whole words using the International Phonetic Alphabet (IPA). The non-English symbols and diacritics expected to be used in the transcription included labiodental stops, bilabial fricatives, unaspirated voiceless stops, wet sounds, and glottal stops. Additional symbols and diacritics were included as needed (see Appendix 1A for recommended extensions of the International Phonetic Alphabet).

3. **Types of Speech Samples.** The clinician's options were to sample spontaneous speech, elicited speech, or a combination of both. Mary's level of development precluded all but spontaneous speech and occasional use of speech imitations (elicited speech).

4. **Elicitation Activities.** The following objects were available to help elicit speech: several simple picture books, a play telephone, a wagon and a toy tricycle, a Mr. Potato head, a doll, blocks, and several big-piece puzzles.

5. **Options for Standardized Assessment Instruments.** None.

6. **Related Assessments.** In addition to the articulation and phonological assessment, the clinician performed a parent interview, a hearing screening, a complete language evaluation, and an oral-mechanism evaluation.

D. Analysis (Chapter 3)

A. The following options were considered (the order of assessments reflects their presentation in Chapter 3 and does not reflect the order in which they were performed):

Severity or intelligibility

Age Norms

Better abilities

Related analyses

1. **Severity or Intelligibility.** The major clinical options were calculation of percentage of development and clinical judgment scales. The clinician selected a clinical judgment scale. The results indicated that Mary was mildly delayed in articulation and phonological development compared to her adjusted chronological age (21 months).

2. **Age Norms.** The major clinical options were analysis of phonetic inventories, error patterns, and consonants.

   a. **Phonetic Inventories.** The clinical options were to use age norms based on either intelligible words or both intelligible and unintelligible words. The former option was selected because Mary's speech appeared largely intelligible. The number and types of consonants in Mary's phonetic inventory approximated those of a child near 16 months of age.

b. **Error Patterns.** The most pervasive error patterns in Mary's speech were Fronting, Stopping, Cluster Reduction, Final Consonant Deletion, Weak Syllable Deletion, and Prevocalic Voicing. Cluster Reduction, Final Cluster Deletion, and Weak Syllable Deletion occurred on nearly 100% of all possible occasions. Fronting, Stopping, and Prevocalic Voicing occurred on 60% of all possible occasions.

c. **Consonants.** Mary's speech contained two established consonants ([b] and [d]) and three emerging consonants ([f], [p], and [k]). [f], [b], [p], and [d] occurred word-initially and [k] occurred word-finally.

3. **Better Abilities.** The clinical options were stimulability, key environments, and key words. Mary was stimulable for [f]. No key environments or key words were found.

4. **Related Analyses.** The clinical options were developmental age, adjusted age, dialect, and acquisition strategies. Mary's developmental age approximated a child of 20–24 months of age. Mary's adjusted age was 21 months. No clinically relevant dialect characteristics were noted in Mary's or her family's speech. The options for acquisition strategies that the clinician considered included regressions, favorite sounds, selectivity, word recipes, homonyms, word-based learning, and gestalt learning. No prominent acquisition strategies were noted.

E. Treatment (Chapter 4)

Mary was accepted into treatment in an early intervention program.

1. **Purpose.** Articulation and phonological care focused on facilitating the acquisition of sounds in specific words.

2. **Long-term Goals.** The long-term goal of treatment for Mary was for articulation and phonological development to be

commensurate with her adjusted chronological age. A second long-term treatment goal was to facilitate parent education and training.

3. **Short-term Goals.** The clinical options were reduction in homonyms, reduction in variability, maximization of established speech abilities, and elimination of errors affecting classes of sounds (either distinctive feature or error pattern approach). Mary's speech did not contain a lot of homonyms or variability, so goals directed to remediating those areas were not considered further. Mary also did not appear stalled in development according to parental report, only somewhat slower compared to other children of her age, so maximization of established speech abilities was not considered as a possible short-term treatment goal. The remaining option, elimination of errors affecting sound classes, was selected as Mary's short-term goal. An error pattern approach was selected. Prevocalic Voicing, Stopping, and Fronting were selected as the first foci of treatment because Mary had demonstrated some ability to produce sounds affected by these errors.

4. **Selecting Treatment Targets.** The clinical options were to select treatment targets that occurred in key words or were emerging, stimulable, or both. When considering the latter two options (emerging and stimulable), the clinician gave greatest priority to potential treatment targets that were both emerging and stimulable but did not exclude potential treatment targets that met one or the other criterion.

5. **Most and Least Knowledge Methods.** The options the clinician considered were to select treatment targets most like the client's existing sounds (a traditional most knowledge method) or treatment targets least like the client's existing sounds (least knowledge method). The clinician selected the latter option, hoping this would improve the likelihood that Mary would generalize treatment success to untreated sounds. For this reason, [k] was considered a preferred treatment target compared to [p], because [k] differed from Mary's established consonants in both place and voicing, whereas [p] differed from Mary's established consonants only in voicing. Similarly, [f] was considered a preferred treatment target compared to both [k] and [p], because [f] differed from Mary's established consonants in place, manner, and voicing.

6. **Number of Treatment Targets.** The clinical options were to train wide or train deep. The clinician selected training wide (three or more treatment targets) to maximize Mary's opportunities to generalize treatment success to untreated sounds.

7. **Changing Treatment Targets.** The clinician's options were flexibility, time, and percentage. The clinician selected time, because it appeared best-suited to Mary's level of cognitive development. If, however, Mary had appeared to have attention difficulties or more substantive cognitive limitations, the clinician would likely have selected flexibility.

8. **Linguistic Level to Introduce Treatment Targets.** The clinical options are isolated sounds, nonsense syllables, words, and phrases. Mary's level of development precluded all but words from consideration.

F. Administrative Decisions (Chapter 4)

The administrative decisions involved session length, group or individual care, length of individual treatment activities, and types of activities. The clinician elected to provide treatment as part of an early intervention program three times a week. Group sessions typically lasted approximately 45 minutes, 15 minutes of which were devoted primarily to speech and language development. The length of specific activities in treatment sessions was approximately 5 minutes. Activities were presented in a therapeutic play format.

G. Facilitative Techniques (Chapter 5)

The clinician's options for facilitative techniques were bombardment, parallel talk, expansions, touch cues, modeling, and requests for confirmation or clarification.

Treatment was organized in cycles. The first cycle provided treatment for Fronting, Prevocalic Voicing, and Stopping. In principle, up to one half of the sounds in an error pattern received treatment. In practice, the requirements of stimulability or emerging sounds restricted the treatment targets to far fewer sounds. The first cycle continued until all treatment targets had received remediation. Error patterns were treated in subsequent cycles until Mary's production of sounds within the error pattern was commensurate with that of children of her adjusted chronological age. Additional error patterns were added to treatment as ongoing evaluation indicated additional sounds in the error patterns became either stimulable or emerging.

Prior to beginning treatment on an error pattern, the clinician and Mary's parents identified the words that were to receive special attention during treatment and at home. Treatment for [k], for example, began with bombardment with approximately 10 words beginning with [k]. Included among these words were three words that were also to be facilitated at home. The words referred to objects that the clinician named as they were drawn out of a "magic box." Production activities involved therapeutic play during which the primary facilitative technique was expansion, supplemented by parallel talk, modeling, and requests for confirmation or clarification. Touch cues for treatment sounds were also introduced. The session concluded with a bombardment activity similar to the one at the beginning of the session.

H. Assessing Clinical Progress (Chapter 4)

The clinician's primary options were pre- and post-tests, ongoing information gathering, and parent questionnaires. The clinician elected to use a clinical judgment of severity and the word lists presented during treatment as pre- and post-tests. A parent interview designed to ascertain both the family's knowledge of speech development and their degree of satisfaction with Mary's progress in speech development was also undertaken. Results of post-testing indicated fair clinical progress; Mary's family demonstrated increased knowledge of speech development in response to questions asked by the clinician and they expressed satisfaction with their daughter's clinical progress.

Vowels

Research on vowels is still in the early stages (Bleile, 1988; Davis & MacNeilage, 1990; Otomo & Stoel-Gammon, 1992; Pollock & Keiser, 1990). Nonetheless, the time may come in a few years when clinical investigators are ready to address such fundamental issues such as: Should vowel errors be remediated, or is it better to continue to focus on consonant acquisition and allow vowel acquisition to proceed without intervention? If vowel errors are to be remediated, further questions arise: Are touch cues effective remediation techniques? Are there direct instruction techniques that facilitate vowel acquisition? What type of language or metaphors are effective in talking about vowels with children? Are indirect facilitative techniques effective in remediating vowel errors?

IV. MAJOR CARE OPTIONS FOR CLIENTS IN STAGE 3

A. The Client: Robert

Robert was born after an unremarkable pregnancy and delivery. Robert's medical and developmental history were similarly unremarkable; however Robert's mother noted that "Kids have trouble understanding his speech, although I usually know what he means." Robert was referred to a speech-language clinician when he entered preschool at 4 years of age.

B. Legal Basis of Care (Chapter 1)

Robert was eligible to be considered for intervention under provisions of PL 94–142, which mandates free and appropriate education to all children with handicaps aged 3 through 21 years. Appropriate education includes a thorough assessment to determine the nature and degree of disability, education tailored to the individual needs of children, placement in the least restrictive environment, and the provision of supplementary services to help ensure success for each child.

C. Assessment (Chapter 2)

The assessment consisted of three steps: initial observation, collection of the speech sample, and hypothesis testing. The initial observation occurred during the parent interview while the clinician spoke with Robert's mother. For the elicitation portion of the assessment, the clinician presented Robert with pictures from a published assessment instrument and transcribed Robert's speech during naming activities while playing. The hypothesis testing occurred during the initial assessment and the beginning of one subsequent treatment session. The clinician concentrated on Robert's most prevalent error patterns using the error probes presented in Appendix 2C. Due to time limitations, error patterns that appeared relatively minor (e.g., deletion of [d] in "window") were set aside for later consideration.

1. **Sample Size.** The clinician's option was to collect between 50 to 100 utterances either in the form of sentences, single words, or a combination of both.

2. **Transcription System.** The clinician transcribed whole words using the International Phonetic Alphabet (IPA). The non-English symbols and diacritics expected to be used in the transcription of Robert's speech included labiodental stops, unaspirated voiceless stops, wet sounds, glottal stops, [w] coloring of [r], lisping, lateralization, and bladed productions of [s] and [z]. Additional symbols and diacritics were included as needed (see Appendix 1A for recommended extensions of the International Phonetic Alphabet).

3. **Types of Speech Samples.** The clinician's options were to obtain samples of spontaneous speech, elicited speech, or a combination of both. During the initial observation, the clinician noted errors occurring in Robert's spontaneous speech. The major portion of the speech sample, however, was derived from single words.

4. **Elicitation Activities.** The clinician selected elicitation activities from those listed in Chapter 2.

5. **Options for Standardized Assessment Instruments.** The following published instruments offered options to assess error patterns:

   The Assessment of Phonological Processes — Revised

   Bankson-Bernthal Test of Phonology

   Compton-Hutton Phonological Assessment

   The Khan-Lewis Phonological Analysis

Natural Process Analysis

Phonological Process Analysis

The clinician elected to use pictures from the *Bankson-Bernthal Test of Phonology* to assist in the collection of the speech sample. Nonstandardized techniques were used to analyze the speech sample.

6. **Related Assessments.** In addition to the articulation and phonological assessment, the clinician performed a parent interview, a hearing screening, a complete language evaluation, and an oral-mechanism evaluation.

D. Analysis (Chapter 3)

The following assessment options were considered (the order of assessments reflects their presentation in Chapter 3 and does not reflect the order in which they were performed):

Severity or intelligibility

Age norms

Better abilities

Related analyses

1. **Severity or Intelligibility.** The major clinical options were percentage of consonants correct, calculation of percentage of development, and clinical judgment scales of severity and intelligibility. The clinician selected a clinical judgment scale of severity. The clinician's judgment was that Robert was moderately delayed in articulation and phonological development compared to his chronological age.

2. **Age Norms.** The major clinical options were phonetic inventories, error patterns, and consonant and consonant clusters.

   a. **Phonetic Inventories.** This analysis was not performed because Robert's articulation and phonological development proved more advanced than that of clients who typically benefit from analysis of phonetic inventories.

b. **Error Patterns.** The results of the error probes indicated the following error patterns: Fronting, Cluster Reduction, Final Consonant Deletion, and Stopping. Robert's speech was largely restricted to syllables that were V, CV, and VCV. Robert's consonants were mainly stops and glides. The analysis of the error probes indicated that Fronting occurred on 3 out of 10 words (30%), Cluster Reduction occurred on 9 out of 10 words (90%), and Final Consonant Devoicing and Stopping occurred on 4 out of 10 words (40%).

c. **Consonants and Consonant Clusters.** The consonants and consonant clusters that Robert produced correctly were similar to those of a child near 3 years of age.

3. **Better Abilities.** The clinical options were stimulability, key environments, and key words. The clinical options for stimulability testing were sound probes (Appendix 2B), error probes (Appendix 2C), or stimulability probes (Appendix 3O). The clinician selected the error probes, because these probes had already been used with Robert and, thus, were readily available. Robert was found to be stimulable for [k], [f], and [ʃ] and word-final [d]. The analysis revealed no key environments and several key words.

4. **Related Analyses.** The clinical options were acquisition strategies, developmental age, and dialect. The acquisition strategies and developmental age analyses were not performed because Robert's articulation and phonological development was beyond that of clients who benefit most from acquisition strategy analyses, and results of the language assessment indicated age-appropriate abilities in language comprehension. Robert's family spoke Hawaiian Creole. The dialect assessment (see Appendix 3S) indicated pronunciation of [t] and [d] for interdental fricatives. This was not considered evidence of an articulation and phonological disorder.

E. Treatment (Chapter 4)

Robert was accepted into treatment in a community speech-language program. Because the clinical options for clients in Stages 2 and 3 are generally similar, this section is more abbreviated than previous sections.

1. **Purpose.** Articulation and phonological care focused on eliminating errors affecting classes of sounds.

2. **Long-term Goals.** The long-term treatment goal for Robert was for articulation and phonological development to be commensurate with his chronological age. A second long-term treatment goal was to facilitate parent education and training.

3. **Short-term Goals.** If Robert had been either a younger preschooler or a child with a more severe articulation and phonological disability, the treatment options would have been the same as for Mary (reduction in homonyms, reduction in variability, maximization of established speech abilities, and elimination of errors affecting classes of sounds). The option for short-term goals for clients of Robert's age and general level of disability was elimination of error affecting classes of sounds. The clinical options were to utilize either a distinctive feature or an error pattern approach. The clinician chose an error pattern approach. The first error patterns selected for treatment were Fronting, Final Consonant Devoicing, and Stopping. Consonant Cluster Reduction was not selected as an early short-term treatment goal because Robert displayed limited success producing sounds affected by that error.

4. **Selecting Treatment Targets.** The clinical options were to select treatment targets that were in key words or that were emerging, stimulable, or both. The clinician elected to treat key words and treatment targets that were both emerging and stimulable, but did not exclude potential treatment targets that met one or the other criteria.

5. **Most and Least Knowledge Methods.** The options that the clinician considered were to select treatment targets most like the client's existing sounds (most knowledge method) or treatment targets least like the client's existing sounds (least knowledge method). The clinician selected the latter option, hoping this would improve the likelihood that Robert would generalize treatment success to untreated sounds.

6. **Number of Treatment Targets.** The clinical options were to train wide or train deep. The clinician selected training wide (three or more treatment targets) to maximize Robert's opportunities to generalize treatment success to untreated sounds.

7. **Changing Treatment Targets.** The clinician's options were flexibility, time, and percentage. Time is an appropriate criterion for changing targets with the vast majority of clients in Stage 3. Those who lack the cognitive and attention abilities needed for a time criterion might be provided treatment using the flexible approach described for Bill and Mary. More advanced clients in Stage 3 with good attention skills may be provided treatment using a percentage criteria. The clinician selected a time criterion for Robert.

8. **Linguistic Level to Introduce Treatment Targets.** The clinical options are isolated sounds, nonsense syllables, words, and phrases. The clinician selected the word level to help facilitate generalization to other settings and persons.

F. Administrative Decisions (Chapter 4)

The administrative decisions involved session length, group or individual care, length of individual treatment activities, and types of activities. Robert received 30-minute individual sessions 3 times a week. Individual activities in treatment sessions lasted approximately 10 minutes. The types of activities used during treatment were structured play and drill play.

G. Facilitative Techniques (Chapter 5)

A wide range of clinical options were available, including bombardment, metaphors, descriptions and demonstrations, touch cues, word pairs, techniques to facilitate syllables and words, and facilitative talk (parallel talk, expansions, modeling, and requests for confirmation or clarification).

Treatment was organized in cycles. The error patterns treated in the first cycle were Fronting, Final Consonant Devoicing, and Stopping. From two sounds up to one half of the sounds in an error pattern received treatment in each cycle. When a new treatment target was introduced (e.g., [f]), the client and clinician negotiated to find a metaphor and a touch cue for [f]. Simple descriptions and demonstrations of [f] were also provided.

At the beginning of each session, Robert was bombarded with words containing the treatment target. During the session, Robert and the clinician engaged in structured play and drill play using word pairs, "talk over" games, and key words to focus on perceptual and production aspects of the treatment target. The clinician used facilitative talk techniques during both perceptual and production activities and during the "play break." The session concluded with auditory bombardment and a review of "what we have learned about our sound today." A home program for Robert's family was included as part of treatment to facilitate generalization to the home and other persons.

H. Assessing Clinical Progress (Chapter 4)

The clinician's primary options were pre- and post-tests, ongoing information gathering, and parent questionnaires. The clinician elected to use a clinical judgment of severity and the probes of error patterns (Appendix 2C) as pre- and post-tests. A parent interview designed to ascertain both the family's knowledge of speech development and their degree of satisfaction with Robert's progress in speech development was also undertaken. Results of the post-tests indicated excellent clinical progress. Like Mary's family, Robert's family demonstrated increased knowledge of speech development in response to questions asked by the clinician and they expressed satisfaction with their child's clinical progress.

Language

Approximately 75% to 85% of children with articulation and phonological disorders also experience difficulties in language development (Paul & Shriberg, 1982; Shriberg & Kwiatkowski, 1988). Several clinical investigators have asked whether it is possible that focusing on language goals will also have a positive effect on a client's articulation and phonological development. In a 1990 study, Hoffman and his colleagues found that two 4-year-old children with articulation and phonological disorders showed comparable improvement when treated using either word pairs or an indirect language approach involving the clients' production of narratives (Hoffman, Norris, & Monjure, 1990). What

continued

---

is interesting about these results is that the clients' articulation and phonological development improved during the narrative task, even though they received no direct training on speech (Norris & Hoffman, 1993). More recently, however, a study of 26 preschool-aged clients failed to find that facilitating language goals had an effect on articulation and phonological development (Fey, Cleave, Ravida, Long, Dejmal, & Easton, 1994). This suggests that an indirect approach to treating articulation and phonological disorders may not be applicable to all clients. Perhaps importantly, the children studied by Fey et al. (1994) appeared more severely affected in articulation and phonological development than those treated successfully by Hoffman, Norris, and Monjure (1990).

V. MAJOR CARE OPTIONS FOR CLIENTS IN STAGE 4

A. The Client: James

James' medical history was remarkable for frequent illnesses during the first year of life. One of these resulted in a hospitalization for failure to thrive. James' developmental history was remarkable for the presence of speech and language delays during preschool and early grade school years. Intervention was provided, and James' language problem appeared to be remediated by the end of the 1st grade. In 3rd grade, when James' class began reading for comprehension, it was discovered that James experienced a learning disability. James was referred by his regular teacher for a re-evaluation of speech when he was 9 years of age. The reason for the referral was described as, "James has trouble with some sounds. He gets some teasing when he says things like 'wabbit' for 'rabbit.' "

B. Legal Basis of Care (Chapter 1)

Like Robert, James was eligible to be considered for intervention under provisions of PL 94–142, which mandates free and appropriate education to all children with handicaps aged 3 through 21 years. Appropriate education includes a thorough assessment to determine the nature and degree of disability, education tailored to the individual needs of children, placement in the least restrictive environment, and the provision of supplementary services to help ensure success for each child.

Differential Diagnosis

Would treatment improve if clinicians could make clear differential diagnoses between articulation and phonological disorders? Should a client with an articulation disorder, for example, receive a treatment specifically designed to remediate problems in the speech motor component, and should a client with a phonological disorder receive a different treatment program designed specifically to remediate the phonological component of a language disorder? Or are articulation and phonology so closely interrelated that treatment for both disorders would be the same no matter what the source of the client's problem? Clearly, the conceptual difference between language (phonology) and speech motor control (articulation) is significant, but whether this distinction will lead to differences in treatment remains to be determined.

C. Assessment (Chapter 2)

The assessment consisted of three steps: initial observation, collection of the speech sample, and hypothesis testing. The initial observation occurred during the first minutes after James entered the treatment room while he and the clinician spoke together about James' classes, favorite subjects, and favorite activities. For the elicitation portion of the assessment, the clinician asked James to name pictures from a published assessment instrument. For the hypothesis testing portion of the assessment, the clinician asked James to name words that contained sounds James had produced in error during the initial observation and elicitation. Stimulability testing and brief trials using phonetic placement and shaping techniques were also attempted. The word lists used during hypothesis testing are contained Appendix 2B, and the phonetic placement and shaping techniques are described in Chapter 5.

1. **Sample Size.** The clinician's option was to collect 50 to 100 utterances in the form of sentences, single words, or a combination of both. The major portion of the speech sample was single words.

2. **Transcription System.** The clinician began by transcribing the entire word but changed to simply transcribing sounds in error after it became clear that James' errors involved late-acquired consonants and consonant clusters. The clinician transcribed using the International Phonetic Alphabet (IPA). The non-English symbols and diacritics expected to be used in the transcription of James' speech included [w]-coloring of [r] and lisped, lateralized, and bladed production of [s] and [z]. Additional symbols and diacritics were included as needed. (See Appendix 1A for recommended extensions of the International Phonetic Alphabet.)

3. **Types of Speech Samples.** The clinician's options for speech samples were spontaneous speech, elicited speech, or a combination of both. During the initial observation the clinician noted errors occurring in James' spontaneous speech; the major portion of the speech sample, however, consisted of single words.

4. **Elicitation Activities.** The clinician selected elicitation activities from those listed in Chapter 2.

5. **Options for Standardized Assessment Instruments.** The following published instruments offer options to assess individual consonants and consonant clusters:

Arizona Articulation Proficiency Scale

Clinical Probes of Articulation Consistency

A Deep Test of Articulation

Edinburgh Articulation Test

Fisher-Logemann Test of Articulation Competence

Goldman-Fristoe Test of Articulation

Photo Articulation Test

The Templin-Darley Tests of Articulation

Test of Minimal Articulation Competence

Test of Phonological awareness

Weiss Comprehensive Articulation Test

The clinician elected to use the picture cards from the *Photo Articulation Test* for the collection of the speech sample. Non-standardized techniques were used to analyze the speech sample.

6. **Related Assessments.** In addition to the articulation and phonological assessment, the clinician performed a parent interview, a hearing screening, a complete language evaluation, and an oral-mechanism evaluation.

D. Analysis (Chapter 3)

The following assessment options were considered (the order of assessments reflects their presentation in Chapter 3 and not the order in which they were performed):

Severity or intelligibility

Age norms

Better abilities

Related analyses

1. **Severity or Intelligibility.** The major clinical options were calculation of percentage of development, ACI, and clinical judgment scales of severity and intelligibility. The clinician selected a clinical judgment scale of severity. The clinician's judgment was that James was mildly delayed in articulation and phonological development compared to his chronological age peers.

2. **Age Norms.** The clinical option was consonants and consonant clusters. James produced the following errors: lateral [s] for [s] and [w] for [r]. The sounds [s] and [r] are typically acquired near 3;6 by 50% of children, and [s] is acquired near 5,0 by 75% of children and [r] is acquired near 6;0 by 75% of children.

3. **Better Abilities.** The clinical options were stimulability, key environments, key words, and phonetic placement and shaping. The clinical options for stimulablity testing were the

sound probes (Appendix 2B) and stimulability probes (Appendix 3O). The clinician selected the sound probes, because these probes were already being used with James and, thus, were readily available. James was found to be stimulable for [r], but not for lateral [s]. No key environments or key words were discovered. Both [r] and lateral [s] appeared to be responsive to shaping and phonetic placement techniques.

4. **Related Analyses.** The clinical options were developmental age and dialect. James' developmental level was found to approximate a child about 8 years of age. James spoke a variety of American English that did not require special assessment.

E. Treatment (Chapter 4)

James was accepted into the speech-language treatment program in his school.

1. **Purpose.** Articulation and phonological care focused on eliminating errors affecting late-acquired consonants, consonant clusters, and unstressed syllables in more difficult multisyllabic words.

2. **Long-term Goals.** The long-term treatment goals for James were for articulation and phonological development to be commensurate with his developmental age and to eliminate speech characteristics that affected his quality of life. A concomitant long-term treatment goal was to facilitate parent education.

3. **Short-term Goals.** The options for short-term goals were consonants and consonant clusters in error.

4. **Selecting Treatment Targets.** The clinical options were to select treatment targets in key words, or treatment targets that were emerging, stimulable, or capable of being produced using either phonetic placement or shaping techniques. The clinician selected to treat [r], both because it was stimulable and because the [w] for [r] error led to James being teased. The clinician also elected to treat lateral [s], because a quick session of trial therapy indicated that James could produce [s] through phonetic placement and shaping techniques.

5. **Most and Least Knowledge Methods.** The options the clinician considered were to select treatment targets most like the client's existing sounds (most knowledge method) or treatment targets least like the client's existing sounds (least knowledge method). Only the former option was relevant due to the small number of errors in James' speech.

6. **Number of Treatment Targets.** The clinical options were to train wide or train deep. Perforce, the clinician selected training deep (one or two treatment targets).

7. **Changing Treatment Targets.** The clinician's options were flexibility, time, and percentage. The clinician selected percentage, because James had the attention skills and other cognitive abilities to make this approach feasible.

8. **Linguistic Level to Introduce Treatment Targets.** The clinical options were isolated sounds, nonsense syllables, words, and phrases. The clinician selected the word level to facilitate generalization to other settings and persons. Isolated sounds and nonsense syllables were utilized as prompts when James experienced failure at the word level.

F. Administrative Decisions (Chapter 4)

The administrative decisions involved session length, group or individual care, length of individual treatment activities, and types of activities. Ideally, James would have received individual sessions four to five times a week. Due to caseload size, James received treatment twice a week, once in a group and the other time individually. The group sessions lasted approximately 45 minutes, and the individual session lasted approximately 30 minutes. Activities in both group and individual sessions lasted approximately 10 to 15 minutes. The format for activities was drill play.

G. Facilitative Techniques (Chapter 5)

The options included the full range of facilitative techniques discussed in Chapter 5 (bombardment, metaphors, descriptions and demonstrations, touch cues, word pairs, techniques to facilitate syllables and words, facilitative talk (parallel talk, expansions, modeling, and requests for confirmation or clarification), and direct instruction techniques (phonetic placement and shaping). Touch cues and facilitative talk were not selected, because the clinician judged that James would find them "immature."

Each treatment target received treatment until it was produced correctly 75% of the time in spontaneous speech, after which the next treatment target received attention until the same percentage criterion was reached. When a new treatment target was introduced (e.g., [r]), the client and clinician negotiated to find a metaphor, and James was taught basic perceptual and production characteristics of the treatment target using simple descriptions and demonstrations. Games involving word pairs and stories containing [r] were used to help James identify the occurrence of the treatment target.

At the beginning of each session, the clinician and James briefly reviewed the previous session. Next, the clinician engaged James in production activities selected from the following list: phonetic placement and shaping games, games involving word pairs, barrier games, and storytelling activities involving names and objects containing the treatment target. During treatment breaks, the clinician listened to observe James' progress in producing the treatment target in spontaneous speech. The session concluded with a brief review of the day's progress. A home program for James' family was included as part of the treatment to facilitate generalization to the home and other persons.

H. Assessing Clinical Progress (Chapter 4)

The clinician's primary options were pre- and post-tests, ongoing information gathering, and parent and client questionnaires. The clinician elected to use a clinical judgment of severity and the error lists presented during treatment as pre- and post-tests. A parent interview designed to ascertain both the family's knowledge of speech development and their degree of satisfaction with James' progress in speech development was also undertaken. Results of the post-tests indicated good clinical progress. James' family demonstrated increased knowledge of speech development in response to questions asked by the clinician and they expressed satisfaction with their son's clinical progress.

REFERENCES

Anthony, A., Bogle, D., Ingram, T., & McIsaac, M. (1971). *The Edinburgh Articulation Test*. Edinburgh, UK: Churchill Livingstone.

Bankson, N., & Bernthal, J. (1990). *Quick Screen of Phonology*. Chicago: Riverside Press.

Bankson, N., & Bernthal, J. (1990). *Bankson-Bernthal Test of Phonology*. Chicago: Riverside Press.

Batshaw, M. (1992). *Children with disabilities: A medical primer* (3rd ed.). Baltimore, MD: Paul H. Brookes.

Bernhardt, B. (in press). Phonological intervention techniques for syllable and word structure development. *Clinics in Communication Disorders*

Bernhardt, B., & Gilbert, J. (1992). Applying linguistic theory to speech-language pathology: The case of non-linear phonology. *Clinical Linguistics and Phonetics, 6,* 123–145.

Bernhardt, B., & Stoel-Gammon, C. (in press). Nonlinear phonology: Introduction and clinical application. *Journal of Speech and Hearing Research.*

Bernthal, J., & Bankson, N. (1993). *Articulation and phonological disorders*. Englewood Cliffs, NJ: Prentice-Hall.

Blache, S. (1989). A distinctive feature approach. In N. Creaghead, P. Newman, & W. Secord (Eds.), *Assessment and remediation of articulatory and phonological disorders* (pp. 361–382). Columbus, OH: Charles E. Merrill.

Bleile, K. (1988). A note on vowel patterns in two normally developing children. *Clinical Linguistics and Phonetics, 3,* 203–212.

Bleile, K. (1991a). Communication disorders. In M. Batshaw, *Your child has a disability: A complete sourcebook of daily and medical care* (pp. 139–151). Boston, MA: Little, Brown.

Bleile, K. (1991b). *Child phonology: A book of exercises for students*. San Diego, CA: Singular Publishing Group.

Bleile, K. (Ed.). (1993a). *The care of children with long-term tracheostomies*. San Diego, CA: Singular Publishing Group.

Bleile, K. (1993b). Children with long-term tracheostomies. In K. Bleile (Ed.), *The care of children with long-term tracheostomies* (pp. 3–19). San Diego, CA: Singular Publishing Group.

Bleile, K. (in press). Infants and toddlers. In L. McCormick, R. Schiefelbusch, & D. From-Loeb (Eds.), *Language intervention in inclusive settings: An introduction* (3rd ed.). New York: Allyn & Bacon.

Bleile, K., & Hand, L. (in press). Metalinguistics. *Journal of Clinical Linguistics and Phonetics.*

Bleile, K., & Miller, S. (1994). Toddlers with medical needs. In J. Bernthal & N. Bankson (Eds.), *Articulatory and phonological disorders in special populations* (pp. 81–100). New York: Thieme.

Bleile K., Stark R., & Silverman McGowan, J. (1993). Evidence for the relationship between babbling and later speech development. *Clinical Linguistics and Phonetics, 7,* 319–337.

Bleile, K., & Tomblin, J. (1991). Regressions in the phonological development of two children. *Journal of Psycholinguistic Research, 20,* 483–499.

Bleile, K., & Wallach, H. (1992). A sociolinguistic investigation of the speech of African American preschoolers. *American Journal of Speech-Language Pathology, 1,* 54–62.

Blodgett, E., & Miller, V. (1989). *Easy Does It for Phonology.* East Moline, IL: Lingui-Systems.

Bradley, D. (1989). A systematic multiple-phoneme approach. In. N. Creaghead, P. Newman, & W. Secord (Eds.), *Assessment and remediation of articulatory and phonological disorders* (pp. 305–322). Columbus, OH: Charles E. Merrill.

Bricker, P., Bailey, E., & Bruder, M. (1984). The efficacy of early intervention and the handicapped infant: A wise or wasted resource? In M. Wolraich & D. Routh (Eds.), *Advances in developmental and behavioral pediatrics* (pp. 373–423). Greenwich, NY: JAI Press.

Bruner, J. (1983). *Child's talk: Learning to use language.* New York: W. W. Norton.

Carrow, E. (1974). *Austin Spanish Articulation Test.* Austin, TX: Teaching Resources Corporation.

Cheng, L. (1987). *Assessing Asian language performance: Guidelines for evaluating limited-English-proficient students.* Rockville, MD: Aspen.

Cole, L., & Taylor, O. (1990). Performance of working class African American children on three tests of articulation. *Language, Speech, and Hearing Services in Schools, 21,* 171–176.

Compton, A., & Hutton, S. (1978). *Compton-Hutton Phonological Assessment.* San Francisco: Carousel House.

Costello, J., & Onstein, J. (1976). The modification of multiple articulation errors based on distinctive feature theory. *Journal of Speech and Hearing Disorders, 31,* 199–215.

Creaghead, N., Newman, P., & Secord, W. (1989). *Assessment and remediation of articulatory and phonological disorders.* Columbus, OH: Charles E. Merrill.

Curtiss, S., Katz, W., & Tallal, P. (1992). Delay versus deviance in the language acquisition of language-impaired children. *Journal of Speech and Hearing Research, 35,* 373–383.

Davis, B., & MacNeilage, P. (1990). Acquisition of correct vowel production: A quantitative case study. *Journal of Speech and Hearing Research, 33,* 16–27.

Dean, E., & Howell, J. (1986). Developing linguistic awareness: A theoretically based approach to phonological disorders. *British Journal of Disorders of Communication, 21,* 223–238.

Dean, E., Howell, J., Hill, A., & Waters, D. (1990). *Metaphon resource pack*. Windsor, UK: NFER-Nelson.

Dean, E., Howell, J., & Waters, D. (1993, November). *Metaphon: An approach to treating children with phonological disorder*. Paper presented to the annual conference of the American Speech-Language-Hearing Association. Anaheim, CA.

Dean, E. Howell, J. Waters, D., & Reid, J. (in press). Metaphon: A metalinguistic approach to the treatment of phonological disorder in children. *Journal of Clinical Linguistics and Phonetics*.

Diedrich, W. (1983). Stimulability and articulation disorders. In J. Locke (Ed.), *Seminars in Speech and Language, 4*.

Dore, J. (1986). The development of conversational competence. In R. Schiefelbusch (Ed.), *Language competence: Assessment and intervention* (pp. 3–59). San Diego, CA: College-Hill Press.

Dunn, L., & Dunn, L. (1981). *Peabody Picture Vocabulary Test — Revised*. Circle Pines, MN: American Guidance Service.

Dyson, A. (1988). Phonetic inventories of 2- and 3-year-old children. *Journal of Speech and Hearing Disorders, 53*, 89–93.

Edwards, M. (1986). *Introduction to applied phonetics*. San Diego, CA: College-Hill Press.

Elbert, M., & Gierut, J. (1986). *Handbook of clinical phonology: Approaches to assessment and treatment*. Austin, TX: Pro-Ed.

Elbert, M., Powell, T., &Swartzlander, R. (1991). Toward a technology of generalization: How many examples are sufficient? *Journal of Speech and Hearing Research, 34*, 81–87.

Elbert, M., Rockman, B., & Saltzman, D. (1980). *The use of minimal pairs in articulation training*. Austin, TX: Exceptional Resources.

Elbert, M., Rockman, B., & Saltzman, D. (1982). *The sourcebook: A phonemic guide to monosyllabic English words*. Austin, TX: Exceptional Resources.

Fairbanks, G. (1960). *Voice and articulation drill book*. New York: Harper & Row.

Ferguson, C., & Farwell, C. (1975). Words and sounds in early language acquisition: English initial consonants in the first fifty words. *Language, 51*, 419–439.

Ferguson, C., & Macken, M. (1983). The role of play in phonological development. In K. Nelson (Ed.), *Child language IV* (pp. 256–282). Hillsdale, NJ: Lawrence Erlbaum.

Fey, M. (1992). Articulation and phonology: Inextricable constructs in speech pathology. *Language, Speech, and Hearing Services in Schools, 23*, 225–232.

Fey, M., Cleave, P., Ravida, A., Long, S., Dejmal, A., & Easton, D. (1994). Effects of grammar facilitation on the phonological performance of children with speech and language impairments. *Journal of Speech and Hearing Research, 37*, 594–607.

Fisher, H., & Logemann, J. (1971). *The Fisher-Logemann Test of Articulation Competence*. Boston, MA: Houghton Mifflin.

Flowers, A. (1990). *The big book of sounds*. Austin, TX: Pro-Ed.

Fluharty, N. (1978). *Speech and Language Screening Test for Preschool Children*. Bingingham, MA: Teaching Resources.

Folkins, J., & Bleile, K. (1990). Taxonomies in biology, phonetics, phonology, and speech motor control. *Journal of Speech and Hearing Disorders, 55*, 596–611.

Fudala, B., & Reynolds, W. (1986). *Arizona Articulation Proficiency Scale*. Los Angeles, CA: Western Psychological Services.

Gierut, J. (1989). Maximal opposition approach to phonological treatment. *Journal of Speech and Hearing Disorders, 54,* 9–19.

Goldman, R., & Fristoe, M. (1986). *Goldman-Fristoe Test of Articulation.* Circle Pines, MN: American Guidance Service.

Goldstein, B. (in press). Spanish phonological development. In H. Kayser (Ed.), *Bilingual speech-language pathology: An Hispanic perspective.* San Diego, CA: Singular Publishing Group.

Gordon-Brannan, M. (1994). Assessing intelligibility: Children's expressive phonologies. *Topics in Language Disorders, 14,* 17–25.

Goswami, U., & Bryant, P. (1990). *Phonological skills and learning to read.* Hillsdale, NJ: Lawrence Erlbaum.

Grunwell, P. (1986). *Phonological Assessment of Child Speech.* Boston: College-Hill Press.

Handler, S. (1993) Surgical management of the tracheostomy. In K. Bleile (Ed.), *The care of children with long-term tracheostomies* (pp. 23–40). San Diego: Singular Publishing Group.

Hodson, B. (1985). *Computer analysis of phonological processes: Version 1.0.* [Computer program]. Danville, IL: Interstate Publishers and Printers.

Hodson, B. (1986a). *Assessment of Phonological Processes — Revised.* Danville, IL: Interstate Publishers and Printers.

Hodson, B. (1986b). *The Assessment of Phonological Processes — Spanish.* San Diego, CA: Los Amigos Association.

Hodson, B. (1989). Phonological remediation: A cycles approach. In N. Creaghead, P. Newman, & W. Secord (Eds.), *Assessment and remediation of articulatory and phonological disorders* (pp. 323–333). Columbus, OH: Charles E. Merrill.

Hodson, B. (1994a). Foreword. *Topics in Language Disorders, 14,* vi–viii.

Hodson, B. (1994b). Becoming intelligible, literate, and articulate. *Topics in Language Disorders, 14,* 1–16.

Hodson, B., & Paden, E. (1991). *Targeting intelligible speech.* Austin, TX: Pro-Ed.

Hoffman, P., Norris, J., & Monjure, J. (1990). Comparison of process targeting and whole language treatments for phonologically delayed preschool children. *Language, Speech, and Hearing Services in Schools, 21,* 102–109.

Hoffman, P., Schuckers, G., & Daniloff, R. (1989). *Children's phonetic disorders: Theory and treatment.* Boston: Little, Brown.

Infant Health and Development Program. (1990). A multisite, randomized trial. *Journal of the American Medical Association, 263,* 3035–3042.

Ingram, D. (1975). Surface contrast in children's speech. *Journal of Child Language, 2,* 287–292.

Ingram, D. (1986). Explanation and phonological remediation. *Child Language Teaching and Therapy, 2,* 1–19.

Ingram, D. (1989). *Phonetic disability in children.* New York: American Elsevier.

Ingram, D. (1994). Articulation testing versus conversational speech sampling: A response to Morrison and Shriberg (1992). *Journal of Speech and Hearing Disorders, 37,* 935–936.

International Clinical Phonetics and Linguistics Association. (1992). Recommended phonetic symbols: Extensions to the IPA. *Clinical Linguistics and Phonetics, 6,* 259–261.

International Clinical Phonetics and Linguistics Association. (1992). The international phonetic alphabet (revised to 1989). *Clinical Linguistics and Phonetics, 6,* 262.

Irwin, J., & Weston, A. (1975). The paired-stimuli monograph. *Acta Symbolica, 6,* 1–76.

Kelman, M., & Edwards, M. (1994). *Phonogroup: A practical guide for enhancing phonological remediation.* Eau Claire, WI: Thinking Publications.

Kent, R., Miolo, G., & Bloedel, S. (1994). Children's Speech Intelligibility Test. *American Journal of Speech-Language Pathology, 3,* 81–95.

Khan, L., & Lewis, N. (1986). *The Khan-Lewis Phonological Analysis.* Circle Pines, MN: American Guidance Service.

Kitley, D., & Buzby-Hadden, J. (1993). Legal rights to education services. In K. Bleile (Ed.), *The care of children with long-term tracheostomies* (pp. 187–202). San Diego, CA: Singular Publishing Group.

Leonard, L. (1985). Unusual and subtle behavior in the speech of phonologically disordered children. *Journal of Speech and Hearing Disorders, 50,* 4–13.

Leinonen-Davies, E. (1988). Assessing the functional adequacy of children's phonological systems. *Clinical Linguistics and Phonetics, 2,* 257–270.

Locke, J. (1983a). Clinical phonology: The explanation and treatment of speech sound disorders. *Journal of Speech and Hearing Disorders, 48,* 339–341.

Locke, J. (1983b). *Phonological acquisition and change.* New York: Academic Press.

Locke, J., & Pearson, D. (1992). Vocal learning and the emergence of phonological capacity: A neurobiological approach. In C. Ferguson, L. Menn, & C. Stoel-Gammon (Eds.), *Phonological development: Models, research, implications* (pp. 91–130). Timonium, MD: York Press.

Long, S., & Fey, M. (1994). *Computerized profiling* [Computer program]. Austin, TX: The Psychological Corporation.

Lowe, R. (1986). *Assessment Link Between Phonology and Articulation.* East Moline, IL: LinguiSystems.

Lowe, R. (1994). *Phonology: Assessment and intervention applications.* Baltimore, MD: Williams & Wilkins.

Lyons, D. (1994). *The effects of Hawaiian Creole on speech and language assessments.* Unpublished master's project, Division of Speech Pathology and Audiology, University of Hawaii, Honolulu.

Maclean, M., Bryant, P., & Bradley, L (1987). Rhymes, nursery rhymes, and reading in early childhood. *Merrill-Palmer Quarterly, 33,* 255–281.

Madison, C. (1979). Articulation stimulability review. *Language, Speech, and Hearing Services in Schools, 10,* 185–190.

Mantovani, J., & Powers, J. (1991). Brain injury in premature infants: Patterns on cranial ultrasound, their relationship to outcome, and the role of developmental intervention in the NICU. *Infants and Young Children, 4,* 20–32.

Mason, R., & Wickwire, N. (1978). Examining for orofacial variations. *Communique, 8,* 2–26.

Masterson, J., & Pagan, F. (1994). *The Macintosh interactive system for phonological analysis* [Computer program] San Antonio, TX: The Psychological Corporation.

Mattes, L. (1993). *Spanish Articulation Measures.* Oceanside, CA: Academic Communication Associates.

McCabe, R., & Bradley, D. (1975). Systematic multiple phonemic approach to articulation therapy. *Acta Symbolica, 6,* 1–18.

McDonald, E. (1964). *Articulation testing and treatment: A sensory-motor approach.* Pittsburgh, PA: Stanwix House.

McDonald, E. (1968). *Screening Deep Test of Articulation.* Pittsburgh, PA: Stanwix House.

McDonald, E. (1964). *A Deep Test of Articulation.* Pittsburgh, PA: Stanwix House.

McReynolds, L., & Bennett, S. (1972). Distinctive feature generalization in articulation training. *Journal of Speech and Hearing Disorders, 37,* 462–470.

McReynolds, L., & Engmann, D. (1975). *Distinctive feature analysis of misarticulations.* Baltimore, MD: University Park Press.

McReynolds, L., & Kearns, K. (1983). *Single-subject experimental designs in communication disorders.* Baltimore, MD: University Park Press.

Menn, L. (1976). *Pattern, control and contrast in beginning speech: A case study in the development of word form and word function.* Unpublished doctoral dissertation, University of Illinois, Champagne-Urbana.

Metz, S. (1993). Ventilator assistance. In K. Bleile (Ed.), *The care of children with long-term tracheostomies* (pp. 41–55). San Diego, CA: Singular Publishing Group.

Miller, J. (1992). Lexical development in young children with Down syndrome. In R. Chapman (Ed.), *Processes in language acquisition and disorders* (pp. 202–216). Philadelphia, PA: Mosby Year Book.

Morrison, J., & Shriberg, L. (1992). Articulation testing versus conversational speech sampling. *Journal of Speech and Hearing Disorders, 35,* 259–273.

Morrison, J., & Shriberg, L. (1992). Response to Ingram letter. *Journal of Speech and Hearing Disorders, 37,* 936–937.

Nemoy, E., & Davis, S. (1954). *The correction of defective consonant sounds.* Magnolia, MA: Expression.

Norris, J., & Hoffman, P. (1993). *Whole language intervention for school-age children.* San Diego, CA: Singular Publishing Group.

Oller, K. (1980). The emergence of the sounds of speech in infancy. In G. Yeni-Komshian, J. Kavanagh, & C. Ferguson (Eds.), *Child phonology: Production* (pp. 93–112). New York: Academic Press.

Oller, K. (1992). Description of infant vocalizations and young child speech: Theoretical and practical tools. *Seminars in Speech and Language, 13,* 178–192.

Oller, K., & Delgado, R. (1990). *Logical International Phonetic Programs* [Computer program]. Miami, FL: Intelligent Hearing Systems.

Otomo, K., & Stoel-Gammon, C. (1992). The acquisition of unrounded vowels in English. *Journal of Speech and Hearing Research, 35,* 604–616.

Parker, F. (1976). Distinctive features in speech pathology: Phonology or phonemics? *Journal of Speech and Hearing Disorders, 41,* 23–39.

Paul, R. (1991). Profiles of toddlers with slow expressive language. *Topics in Language Disorders, 11,* 1–13.

Paul, R., & Shriberg, L. (1982). Associations between phonology and syntax in speech-delayed children. *Journal of Speech and Hearing Research, 25,* 536–547.

Pendergast, K., Dickey, S., Selmar, T., & Soder, A. (1969). *Photo Articulation Test.* Danville, IL: Interstate Publishers and Printers.

Peters, A. (1977). Language learning strategies: Does the whole equal the sum of the parts? *Language, 53,* 560–573.

Peters, A. (1983). *The units of language acquisition*. New York: Cambridge University Press.

Pollock, K., & Keiser, N. (1990). An examination of vowel errors in phonologically disordered children. *Clinical Linguistics and Phonetics, 4,* 161–178.

Powell, T. (1991). Planning for phonological generalization: An approach to treatment target selection. *American Journal of Speech-Language Pathology, 1,* 21–27.

Powell, T., Elbert, M., & Dinnsen, D. (1991). Stimulability as a factor in phonological generalization of misarticulating preschool children. *Journal of Speech and Hearing Research, 34,* 1318–1328.

Proctor, A. (1989). Stages of normal noncry vocal development in infancy: A protocol for assessment. *Topics in Language Disorders, 10,* 26–42.

Ramey, C., & Campbell, F. (1984). Preventive education for high-risk children: Cognitive consequences of the Caroline Abecedarian Project. *American Journal of Mental Deficiency, 88,* 515.

Robb, M., & Bleile, K. (in press). Consonant inventories of young children from 8 to 25 months. *Clinical Linguistics and Phonetics.*

Sander, E. (1972). When are speech sounds learned. *Journal of Speech and Hearing Disorders, 37,* 55–63.

Schoenborn, C., & Marano, M. (1989). *Current estimates from the National Health Interview Survey, United States.* National Center for Health Statistics. Vital and Health Statistics, Series 10, No. 173. DHHS Pub. No. (PHS) 89-1501. Public Heath Service, Washington, DC: Government Printing Office.

Scollon, R. (1976). *Conversations with a one year old: A case study of the developmental foundation of syntax.* Honolulu: The University Press of Hawaii.

Schwartz, R. (1988). Phonological factors in early lexical acquisition. In M. Smith, & J. Locke (Eds.), *The emergent lexicon. The child's development of a linguistic vocabulary* (pp. 185–222). New York: Academic Press.

Schwartz, R. (1992). Nonlinear phonology as a framework for phonological acquisition. In R. Chapman (Ed.), *Processes in language acquisition and disorders* (pp. 108–124). Philadelphia, PA: Mosby Year Book.

Schwartz, R., & Leonard, L. (1982). Do children pick and choose: An examination of phonological selection and avoidance in early lexical acquisition. *Journal of Child Language, 9,* 319–336.

Secord, W. (1981a). *Clinical Probes of Articulation Consistency.* San Antonio, TX: The Psychological Corporation.

Secord, W. (1981b). *Test of Minimal Articulation Competence.* San Antonio, TX: The Psychological Corporation.

Shelton, R. & McReynolds, L. (1979). Functional articulation disorders: Preliminaries to treatment. In N. Lass (Ed.), *Introduction to communication disorders* (pp. 263–310). Englewood Cliffs, NJ: Prentice-Hall.

Shewan, C. (1988). 1988 omnibus survey: Adaptation and progress in times of change. *Asha, 30,* 27–30.

Shriberg, L. (1986). *Programs to examine phonetic and phonologic evaluation records: Version 4.0.* [Computer program]. Hillsdale, NJ: Lawrence Erlbaum.

Shriberg, L. (1993). Four new speech and prosody-voice measures for genetics research and other studies in developmental phonological disorders. *Journal of Speech and Hearing Research, 36,* 105–140.

Shriberg, L., & Kent, R. (1982). *Clinical phonetics*. New York: John Wiley.

Shriberg, L., & Kwiatkowski, J. (1980). *Natural Process Analysis*. New York: John Wiley.

Shriberg, L., & Kwiatowski, J, (1982), Phonological disorders III: A procedure for assessing severity of involvement. *Journal of Speech and Hearing Disorders, 47,* 256–270.

Shriberg, L., & Kwiatkowski, J. (1983). Computer-assisted natural process analysis (NPA): Recent issues and data. In J. Locke (Ed.), *Seminars in Speech and Language, 4,* 397.

Shriberg, L., & Kwiatkowski, J. (1988). A follow-up study of children with phonologic disorders of unknown origin. *Journal of Speech and Hearing Disorders, 53,* 144–155.

Shine, R. (1989). Articulatory production training: A sensory-motor approach. In. N. Creaghead, P. Newman, & W. Secord (Eds.), *Assessment and remediation of articulatory and phonological disorders* (pp. 355–359). Columbus, OH: Charles E. Merrill.

Silverman McGowan, J., Bleile, K., Fus, L., & Barnas, E. (1993). Communication Disorders. In K. Bleile (Ed.), *The care of children with long-term tracheostomies* (pp. 113–140). San Diego: Singular Publishing Group.

Silverman McGowan, J., Kerwin, M., & Bleile, K. (1993). Oral-motor and feeding problems. In K. Bleile (Ed.), *The care of children with long-term tracheostomies* (pp. 89–112). San Diego: Singular Publishing Group.

Slater, S. (1992). Portrait of the professions. *Asha, 34,* 61–65.

Smit, A., Hand, L., Frelinger, J., Bernthal, J., & Byrd, A. (1990). The Iowa articulation norms project and its Nebraska replication. *Journal of Speech and Hearing Disorders, 55,* 779–798.

Snow, C. (1984). Parent-child interaction and the development of communicative ability. In R. Schiefelbusch, & J. Pickar (Eds.), *The acquisition of communication competence* (pp. 69–108). Baltimore, MD: University Park Press.

Snow, C., & Goldfield, B. (1983). Turn the page please: Situation-specific language acquisition. *Journal of Child Language, 10,* 551–569.

Stark, R. (1980). Stages of speech development in the first year of life. In G. Yeni-Komshian, J. Kavanagh, & C. Ferguson (Eds.), *Child phonology: Production* (pp. 73–92). New York: Academic Press.

Stoel-Gammon, C. (1985). Phonetic inventories, 15–24 months: A longitudinal study. *Journal of Speech and Hearing Research, 28,* 505–512.

Stoel-Gammon, C., & Dunn, C. (1985). *Normal and disordered phonology in children*. Baltimore, MD: University Park Press.

Task Force on Health Care. (1993). Task force on health care report. *Asha, 35,* 53–54.

Taylor, O., & Peters-Johnson, C. (1986). Speech and language disorders in Blacks. In O. Taylor (Ed.), *Nature of communication disorders in culturally and linguistically diverse populations*. San Diego: College-Hill Press.

Templin, M., & Darley, F. (1969a). *Templin-Darley Screening Test*. Iowa City: University of Iowa Bureau of Education Research and Service.

Templin, M., & Darley, F. (1969b). *The Templin-Darley Tests of Articulation*. Iowa City: University of Iowa Bureau of Educational Research and Service.

Torgesen, J., & Bryant, B. (1994). *Test of Phonological Awareness*. Austin, TX: Pro-Ed.

Tyler, A. (1993, November). *Different goal attack strategies in phonological treatment*. Paper presented to the annual Conference of the American Speech-Language-Hearing Association, Anaheim, CA.

Tyler, A., Edwards, A., & Saxman, J. (1987). Clinical application of two phonologically based treatment procedures. *Journal of Speech and Hearing Disorders, 52,* 393–409.

U.S. Department of Education. Twelfth annual report to Congress on the implementation of The Education of the Handicapped Act. Washington, DC: Government Printing Office.

Van Riper, C. (1978). *Speech correction: Principles and methods* (6th ed.). Englewood Cliffs, NJ: Prentice-Hall.

Van Riper, C., & Erickson, J. (1968). Predictive Screening Test of Articulation. *Journal of Speech and Hearing Disorders, 34,* 214–219.

Vannucci, J. (1994). *Assessment of vocal behaviors during the first year of life.* Unpublished masters' project, Division of Speech Pathology and Audiology, University of Hawaii, Honolulu.

Vihman, M., Ferguson, C., & Elbert, M. (1986). Phonological development from babbling to speech: Common tendencies and individual differences. *Applied Psycholinguistics, 7,* 3–40.

Walsh, S. (1994). *A resource for treatment of articulatory and phonological disorders: Minimally and maximally contrasting word pairs.* Unpublished masters' project. University of Hawaii, Honolulu.

Waterson, N. (1971). Child phonology: A prosodic view. *Journal of Linguistics, 7,* 179–221.

Webster, P., & Plante, A. (1992). Effects of phonological impairment on word, syllable, and phoneme segmentation and reading. *Language, Speech, and Hearing Services in Schools, 23,* 176–182.

Weiner, F. (1979). *Phonological Process Analysis.* Austin, TX: Pro-Ed.

Weiner, F. (1981). Treatment of phonological disability using the method of meaningful minimal contrast: Two case studies. *Journal of Speech and Hearing Disorders, 46,* 97–103.

Weiner, F. (1986). *Process analysis: Version 2.0* [Computer program]. State College, PA: Parrot Software.

Weiss, C. (1980). *Weiss Comprehensive Articulation Test.* Chicago, IL: Riverside.

Weiss, C., Gordon, M., & Lillywhite, H. (1987). *Clinical management of articulatory and phonologic disorders.* Baltimore, MD: Williams & Wilkins.

White, K., Mastrapierl, M., & Casto, G. (1984). An analysis of special education early childhood projects approved by the joint dissemination review panel. *Journal of the Division of Early Childhood, 9,* 11.

Williams, L. (1991). Generalization patterns associated with training least phonological knowledge. *Journal of Speech and Hearing Research, 34,* 722–723.

Williams, L. (1993). Phonological reorganization: A qualitative measure of phonological improvement. *American Journal of Speech-Language Pathology, 2,* 44–51.

Winitz, H. (1984). *Treating articulation disorders.* Baltimore, MD: University Park Press.

Yavas, M., & Lamprecht, R. (1988). Processes and intelligibility in disordered phonology. *Clinical Linguistics and Phonetics, 2,* 329–345.

Zimmerman, I., Steiner, V., & Pond, R. (1992). *Preschool Language Scale 3.* Columbus, OH: Charles E. Merrill.

INDEX